NutriSearch

Comparative Guide to
Nutritional
Supplements™

for the Americas

NutriSearch

Comparative Guide to

Nutritional Supplements™

for the Americas

BY LYLE MACWILLIAM, MSc, FP

FOR NUTRISEARCH CORPORATION

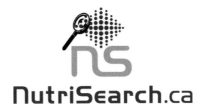

NutriSearch.ca

NUTRISEARCH COMPARATIVE GUIDE TO NUTRITIONAL SUPPLEMENTS FOR THE AMERICAS™

This guide is produced for educational and comparative purposes only. No person should use the information herein for self-diagnosis, treatment, or justification in accepting or declining any medical treatment for any health-related problems. Some medical therapies, including the use of medicines, may be affected by the use of certain nutritional supplements. Therefore, any individual with a specific health problem should seek advice by a qualified medical practitioner before starting a supplementation program. The decision whether to consume any nutritional supplement rests with the individual, in consultation with his or her medical advisor. Furthermore, nothing in this manual should be misinterpreted as medical advice.

This guide is intended to assist in sorting through the maze of nutritional supplements available in the marketplace today. It does not make any health claim. It simply documents recent findings in the scientific literature.

Library and Archives Canada Cataloguing in Publication

MacWilliam, Lyle Dean
[Comparative guide to nutritional supplements]
NutriSearch comparative guide to nutritional supplements
for the Americas / by Lyle MacWilliam, MSc, FP ; for NutriSearch
Corporation.

Includes bibliographical references.
ISBN 978-0-9812840-7-1 (pbk.)

1. Dietary supplements. 2. Dietary supplements--Evaluation.
I. NutriSearch Corporation, issuing body II. Title. III. Title: Comparative
guide to nutritional supplements for the Americas.

RM258.5.M334 2015   615.1   C2015-900824-7

Some say that, in the origin of things,

When all creation started into birth,

The infant elements received a law,

From which they swerve not since; that under force

Of that controlling ordinance they move,

And need not His immediate hand, who first

Prescribed their course, to regulate it now.

~ William Cowper 1731 – 1800
"The Winter Walk at Noon" (excerpt)

Table of Contents

Figures and Tables

ON A PERSONAL NOTE

Since its inaugural publication in 1999, the *Comparative Guide to Nutritional Supplements* has evolved into a recognized standard for the rating of nutritional supplements in the global marketplace. Now in its second decade and previously published in Canada, the United States, Australia, New Zealand, and Mexico, the guide serves as an indispensable tool in helping health-conscious consumers make informed choices. With translations into French, Spanish, Chinese, and Korean, our work at NutriSearch has taken on a global dimension.

In this regard, we are pleased to announce the addition of Colombia, the first country in South America to be added to our growing global roster. To celebrate this event, NutriSearch has created a single guide for the Americas. Based on a compilation of scientific information contained in the 3rd, 4th, and 5th (North American) editions of the *Comparative Guide* and from field research compiled from 2011 to 2014 throughout Canada, the United States, Mexico, and Colombia, the *NutriSearch Comparative Guide to Nutritional Supplements for the Americas* is a comprehensive single-point reference tool for evaluating nutritional supplements within each of these diverse international markets.

The concept for the NutriSearch Comparative Guide series germinated from my work as a consultant for Health Canada during the late 1990s. At that time, I was appointed by The Honourable Allan Rock, Canada's former Minister of Health, as a member of a team of experts charged with developing an innovative regulatory framework for the manufacture and sale of nutritional supplements in the Canadian marketplace. Our report, with all its 51 recommendations accepted by the Canadian Government, called for sweeping changes in the licensing of products and manufacturers that would ensure Canadian consumers access to nutritional products that were safe, effective, and of high quality. During the deliberations of the advisory team and through the writing and development of its final report, it became clear to me that Canadian consumers—and consumers elsewhere—were largely in the dark about how to assess the quality and efficacy of nutritional products. Thus, as a personal mission, I began to explore a means of helping the consumer separate the 'wheat from the chaff' on the question of nutritional quality. The *Comparative Guide to Nutritional Supplements* is the culmination of this effort.

Now in its 5th edition in North America, the *Comparative Guide to Nutritional Supplements* is an independent publication under license to NutriSearch, a Canadian research house specializing in the evaluation of nutritional products in the global marketplace. The research, development, and findings are the sole creative efforts of NutriSearch Corporation and the author.

From its beginnings, the *Comparative Guide to Nutritional Supplements* has employed an analysis model developed from the published recommendations of several recognized nutritional authorities. With each edition of the guide, we have added new recommendations from authorities who have more recently come to the forefront, and we have incorporated recent scientific findings on specific nutrients to provide an increasingly robust model of optimal nutritional supplementation.

In this edition, we incorporate very recent findings on two nutrients whose pivotal roles in cellular nutrition have long been misunderstood and neglected. Vitamin D and iodine are ancient membrane antioxidants. Their evolutionary assimilation into biological systems far predates all but the earliest of life forms; their roles in cellular growth and metabolism are deeply imbedded in the genetic tapestry of our cells. We review the biology of vitamin D and iodine, and we highlight exciting novel scientific discoveries about their importance in optimal health.

This guide is the work of several dedicated people without whom this production would not have been possible. My thanks go to my wife, Arlene, whose research and editing skills and dogged determination to dig out every last product we could find are unmatched; to Gregg Gies for his tireless efforts in conducting our online data search, for his invaluable technical skills in the development, testing, and modification of our analytical model, and for the final creative layout of the guide; to Bryden Derber, who was able to put 'boots on the ground' and dig out hard-to-locate retail products; and to Kathleen Tite and Tammy Simpson, for their valued help in data verification. Lastly, my thanks go to you, the reader, whose financial contribution through the purchase of these guides makes our continued efforts possible.

In summary, the last 15 years I have spent in creating, developing, and writing this guide have truly been a labour of love. As an educator and biochemist whose early research focused on the protective effects of the antioxidant vitamin E, enlightening myself and others on the wisdom of a holistic approach to preventive health—and the importance of supplementation and lifestyle change as components of that paradigm—has been a journey nothing short of a life's mission.

In my travels as author and speaker I have been witness to innumerable personal testimonies regarding the curative powers attributed to optimal nutrition. It's not magic. It's simply Mother Nature at her best—testimony to the fact that, when provided with the proper nutritional tools to do so, the human body has an amazing capacity to heal. It's what Nobel Laureate Linus Pauling called 'orthomolecular medicine'—healing at the *cellular* level.

I hope that the information provided through this guide will enlighten you in your quest for better health.

To your health,

Lyle MacWilliam

January 1st, 2015

Nature composes some of her loveliest poems for the microscope and the telescope.

~Theodore Roszak (1933 - 2011)
Where the Wasteland Ends, 1972

CHAPTER ONE:

FREE RADICALS AND ANTIOXIDANTS

Cells are the building blocks of life, miraculous biochemical factories far more intricate than we can hope to imagine. It is here, within this microscopic world, that the dance of life bursts forth on a scale of complexity that is stunningly inconceivable. Every second, myriad chemical reactions take place in each of our body's trillions of cells, intricately choreographed in a wondrous biochemical symphony.

Life is a constant flow of energy, and it moves in our cells through a steady transfer of electrons from one molecule to the next. When a molecule gives up an electron it is said to be *oxidized;* when it accepts an electron it is *reduced.* This ongoing to and fro of oxidation/reduction, known to biochemists as cellular redox balance, is the chemical 'yin and yang' of life, powering the machinery of the cell through a complex series of reactions called *respiration.*

It begins with a molecule of glucose, the energy source of the cell. Through a series of oxidation/reduction (redox) reactions,

glucose is broken down to its component parts and energy is alternatively released and captured. Throughout this process, electrons move between molecules to the terminal step, where they combine with oxygen and hydrogen to form water.

In simple terms, respiration is nothing more than controlled oxidation or combustion, much like the burning of wood or the rusting of iron. In our cells, however, the process is much more involved: biological catalysts, specialized proteins called enzymes, control each of the many steps along the respiratory pathway. Enzymes allow the 'oxidative fires' of the cell to burn at a much lower temperature, releasing energy in small packets that are captured and stored as adenosine triphosphate (ATP), a form of energy currency used by the cell. The consequence of this biologically controlled oxidation is essentially the same as simple combustion: complex molecules are broken down to water and carbon dioxide.

In cells, the energy released is captured to drive other metabolic processes.

Along the way, some of the electrons exchanged through the individual steps of respiration invariably escape and leak out of the respiratory centres of the cell to react with ambient oxygen, generating toxic oxygen free radicals. It is estimated that two to five percent of the electrons that pass through the cell's respiratory processes are converted to damaging oxygen free radical species.[1] This continuous flux of free radicals generates considerable oxidative stress in human tissues and threatens the integrity of essential biomolecules within the cell.

> The most important medical discovery of the last half-century concerns two substances called 'free radicals' and 'antioxidants.' Free radicals have been linked to (at last count) about 60 diseases. And we now have evidence that antioxidants can stop and (in some instances) even reverse the damage done by free radicals…
>
> ~ Dr Robert D Willix Jr

Free Radicals:

What are they?

Chemically speaking, free radicals are molecules or molecular fragments that have an unpaired electron. Highly unstable and extremely short lived, these chemical intermediates have a lifespan measured in trillionths of a second. Their presence in biological systems was first reported in the early 1960s, when scientists observed exceedingly short-lived events in enzyme-controlled redox reactions, similar to those that take place inside our cells. Because of their unpaired electrons, free radicals are extremely volatile, reacting aggressively with other molecules at the instant of their creation.

Oxidation/reduction, free radicals, unpaired electrons—this sounds like pretty esoteric stuff; but it's not. Life's quintessential paradox is that oxygen, the giver of life, is also our mortal enemy. While oxygen is essential for cellular respiration, its ability to chemically morph into toxic reactive oxygen species (ROS), including superoxide anion ($\cdot O2-$), hydrogen peroxide (H_2O_2) and the damaging hydroxyl radical ($\cdot HO$), lies at the very heart of cellular aging and disease.

Oxygen is not the only molecule to form free radicals. The biological transfer of electrons, common in respiration and other cellular reactions, also generates reactive nitrogen species, including the nitric oxide radical ($NO\cdot$) and the peroxynitrite radical ($ONOO-$).

While endogenous free radical formation is a daily part of the cell's respiratory processes, free radical formation in cells can also be induced through exposure to exogenous agents, such as environmental pollutants, industrial chemicals, agricultural pesticides, cigarette smoke, and radiation. Even vigorous exercise will release a damaging flood of free radicals that can injure your cells if they are not protected.

Damage occurs when the free radical encounters another molecule and seeks out another electron with which to pair its unpaired electron. The free radical rips an electron away from its neighboring molecule, causing the affected molecule to become a free radical itself. The process is repeated, setting up a chemical chain reaction of free radical production. In cells, free radicals produced in such reactions often remove an electron from an important biomolecule, such as an enzyme or functional protein, which cannot function without it. Such an event causes damage to the molecule, and thus to the cell that contains it.

During their fleeting existence, free radicals can inflict considerable harm to the cell's delicate biochemical machinery, punching tiny holes in cell membranes, altering the cell's molecular blueprint, and tearing apart protein and lipid molecules. For cells lacking appropriate defences, these supercharged particles leave a virtual killing field of destruction in their wake—nasty stuff, with nasty consequences for the cell.

Free Radical Theory

The free radical theory of aging states that organisms age because cells accumulate free radical damage over time.[2] The theory was first proposed in the 1950s by biochemist and Professor Emeritus of Medicine, Dr Denham Harman.[3] In 1972, Harman extended the idea to implicate mitochondrial production of reactive oxygen species as the principal mechanism for damage and disease.[4] According to Harman, aging occurs when cells sustain injury from the lifelong and unrelenting attack of free radicals. The carnage inflicted by their uncontrolled assault damages the integrity of important cellular molecules—the proteins, fats, carbohydrates, and nucleic acids of the cell. Over time, the cumulative damage destroys molecular fidelity and cellular function. It then spreads outward, to involve the tissues and organs, accelerating the aging process and ultimately manifesting in some form of degenerative disease.

Investigators have now linked scores of degenerative diseases to free radical-induced oxidative stress. According to Harman, such diseases are not separate entities, but rather different forms of expression of the aging process, influenced by genetic endowment and environmental factors. Today, an estimated 80 to 90% of all degenerative diseases involve some form of free radical activity.

Free radical damage within cells is now linked to a range of disorders, including cardiovascular disease, cancer, arthritis, atherosclerosis, Alzheimer's disease, and diabetes. There is also evidence that some reactive nitrogen species can trigger cell death mechanisms within the body, leading to apoptosis, a form of cellular suicide. Which disease eventually strikes you depends as much on your individual lifestyle and lifelong dietary choices as it does on the roll of the genetic dice cast at your conception.

Nature's Fire Wardens

According to Dr Edward West, [5] "It is essential that in biological oxidation-reduction the transfer [of energy] takes place in a manner that controls the potentially destructive effects of free radical formation and conserves biological function within the cell." The fundamental control mechanisms, referred to by West, lie in the proper functioning of the enzyme

systems needed for these redox reactions to proceed, as well as in the cell's natural defence mechanisms—antioxidants.

Antioxidants are nature's fire wardens, complex molecules that police the chemical processes of the cell and help snuff out the free radicals generated continuously by the cell's activities. As long as we have sufficient antioxidant stores in our cells, the cellular damage can be controlled. However, if we lack sufficient antioxidant reinforcements, cumulative free radical damage will injure the delicate fabric of life. Such oxidative damage is the dark force behind the onset of degenerative disease.[6]

Until the development of Harman's theory, free radicals were thought to exist only outside the body. However, in 1968, work by Harman showed that a small amount of vitamin E added to the diet increased life spans in mice by about five percent.[7] Until then, not much was known about the relevance of vitamin E or other biological antioxidants; science simply did not understand the importance of such molecules in the protection of the cell against oxidative assault. We now know that antioxidants quench the propagation of free radicals in cellular tissues. They do this by either scavenging the unpaired electron from the free radical or by donating an electron to the radical,

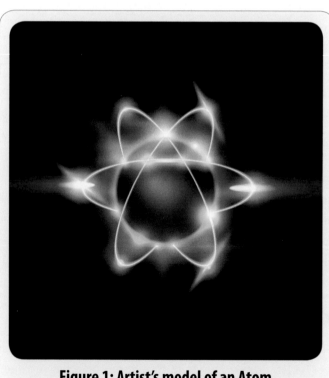

Figure 1: Artist's model of an Atom
Loss of an electron in an atom's outer shell will create a highly unstable and damaging free radical.

rendering the molecule harmless. In the process, the antioxidant, itself, is chemically altered.

The evidence is now irrefutable that the right use of antioxidants can prevent and reverse many forms of cancer, heart disease, atherosclerosis, adult-onset diabetes and a host of other diseases whose primary cause is excess (free radical) oxidation.

~ Dr Michael Colgan

Just like firefighters on the front line, antioxidants work best when they work *together*. Scientists call this phenomenon 'biochemical synergy,' an idiom coined by Dr Richard Passwater, who observed that the effect of the whole is greater than the sum of its parts. This occurs because some antioxidants are regenerated in the presence of other antioxidants, and it is the reason why you should always supplement with a wide spectrum of antioxidants rather than just one. Other antioxidants are converted to entirely different compounds or are excreted from the body. Your body produces some antioxidants; others must be obtained through the diet.

The endogenous antioxidants, those manufactured by the cell, include many of the body's natural enzymes, coenzymes and sulfur-containing molecules, such as glutathione peroxidase, catalase and superoxide dismutase (SOD). The dietary antioxidants include vitamin A (and related carotenoids, including beta carotene), vitamins E and C, iodine, and the myriad bioflavonoids, polyphenols, and sulfur-containing compounds derived from fruits and vegetables. While not themselves antioxidants, many minerals also form vital

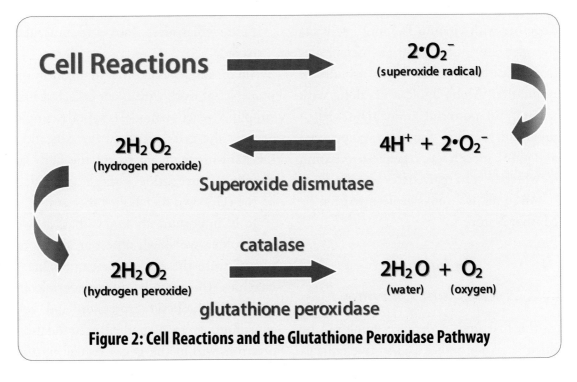

Cell Reactions ➡️ $2 \cdot O_2^-$
(superoxide radical)

$2H_2O_2$ ⬅️ $4H^+ + 2 \cdot O_2^-$
(hydrogen peroxide)

Superoxide dismutase

catalase

$2H_2O_2$ ➡️ $2H_2O + O_2$
(hydrogen peroxide)   (water)   (oxygen)

glutathione peroxidase

Figure 2: Cell Reactions and the Glutathione Peroxidase Pathway

parts of the different antioxidant systems in the body. These include selenium, iron, manganese, copper, and zinc.

Antioxidants also work in different areas of the cell. Vitamin E is the principal antioxidant in the fatty matrix of the cell membrane, quenching free radical-induced lipid peroxidation within the membrane. Iodine, another fat-soluble antioxidant, is active with the cell's membranous structures as well. Vitamin C, on the other hand, is king in the extracellular fluids and works alongside glutathione in the cytoplasm (fluid portion) of the cell. Both vitamin C and vitamin E, along with selenium, enhance the effect of beta carotene. Coenzyme Q_{40} (CoQ_{40}), an enzyme critical to the respiratory process, works deep within the mitochondria (the powerhouses of the cell), assisting in the energy transfer reactions and rejuvenating vitamin E. Together with vitamin E, CoQ_{40} protects the delicate mitochondrial membranes from the relentless oxidative assaults of respiration. Alpha lipoic acid, along with a family of powerful antioxidants called proanthocyanidins, found in grape seed and pine bark extracts, regenerates vitamin C, which in turn rejuvenates vitamin E.

All in all, it's a masterpiece written by Mother Nature.

Endogenous Antioxidant Enzymes

The first line of defence employed by the cells of our bodies against free radicals consists of three protective endogenous (internal) enzymes: superoxide dismutase (SOD), catalase, and glutathione peroxidase. These three antioxidants work together to rid our cells of toxic oxygen free radicals generated through respiration.

Here is how they do their thing (see Figure 2, previous page):

✓ Under the prodding of superoxide dismutase, an important cellular antioxidant enzyme, toxic superoxide radicals produced by the cell's metabolic activities combine with hydrogen ions to form hydrogen peroxide.

✓ To rid itself of hydrogen peroxide, itself a potent free radical generator, the cell enlists the talents of two more antioxidant enzymes, catalase and glutathione peroxidase.

✓ Working together, catalase and glutathione peroxidase split the hydrogen peroxide molecules apart to produce harmless water and molecular oxygen.

There are several other detoxification processes at work within our cells, but this simplified reaction model is a good example of how the cell's principal detoxification mechanisms team up to rid the body of damaging superoxide radicals generated by the cell's own metabolic processes.

It is important to know that, as we grow older, we slowly lose our ability to manufacture these important antioxidant enzymes. This may be due to age-related changes in genetic expression and cell signalling, or to a gradual accumulation of errors within the genes regulating the manufacture of particular antioxidant enzymes. Whatever the cause, once cells can no longer make sufficient amounts of the critical antioxidant enzymes, or they produce faulty copies that don't work very well, free radicals begin to accumulate and oxidative damage accelerates. In simplistic terms, our bodies begin 'rusting away' from within.

We still have much to learn about the precise mechanisms through which antioxidants counteract free radical assaults. Today, largely because of the immense strides made in the mapping of the human genome, it is increasingly recognized that the true nature of antioxidants may not be limited to their ability to act as free radical scavengers. Instead, the *knockout* punch of antioxidants may lie in their recently discovered talents as important cell-signalling molecules, capable of switching on and off a host of genes responsible for the myriad processes controlling redox balance and cellular life itself.

These newest research findings promise to open an entirely new chapter in the unravelling mystery of antioxidants and their central role in protecting the cell and preventing cellular aging and the onset of degenerative disease.

**Don't dig your grave with your
own knife and fork.**

~ Old English Proverb

CHAPTER TWO:

INFLAMMATION ~ EXPLORING THE HIDDEN DANGERS

In April 2005, a paper published in the *Archives of Internal Medicine* revealed startling new findings on the nature of heart disease. The paper, a systematic review on the effect of various fat-reducing agents on heart disease, combined the data from 97 individual clinical trials and compared the reductions in cardiac death rates from various interventions to treat high cholesterol. Mortality data involving 137,000 patients from six types of intervention—including the use of cholesterol-busting drugs, cholesterol-binding resins, high-dose niacin, fish oil supplementation, and dietary change—were compared to data from 139,000 control subjects.

Much to the chagrin of the pharmaceutical industry, the researchers found that the greatest benefit was obtained from *fish oil*, which provided a 23% reduction in the overall risk of death.[1] Conversely, mainstream medicine's weapon of choice, statin drugs, conferred only a 13% reduction in risk. When the risk of death from heart disease alone was examined, fish oil lowered mortality by a whopping 32% compared to 22% from statin drugs. Even more remarkable, fish oil provided this extraordinary protection while exhibiting the *least* ability amongst all forms of intervention to actually lower cholesterol levels.

These findings strongly refute the classic view of heart disease based on the standard model of cholesterol blockage—a model that utterly fails to explain why 70% of heart attacks occur in people with little or no previous arterial blockage. The authors of the study suggest that the protective effect of fish oil must be expressed through a mechanism entirely unrelated to cholesterol levels.

That mechanism rests upon a hypothesis proffered over 150 years ago by the renowned 19th century pathologist, Rudolph Virchow, who proposed that systemic *inflammation* might be the trigger that precipitates a fatal cardiac event. From research conducted since the 1980s, we have now closed the circle to embrace Virchow's original paradigm: cardiovascular disease, the leading cause of preventable death in our modern world, is a bona-fide inflammatory condition.[2]

Heart Disease and Inflammation

Harvard cardiologist Paul Ridker has come to view heart disease as an inflammatory process that is similar to rheumatoid arthritis. Based on several studies that suggest up to 25 million Americans with normal cholesterol have markedly higher risks for heart attack due to systemic inflammation,[3-5] Ridker believes that chronic inflammation is implicated in no less than 50% of diagnosed heart disease cases.

Ridker's research has identified C-reactive protein (CRP) as a principal clinical marker for systemic inflammation. Produced by the liver and the specialized cells that line the arterial walls, levels of this cellular signalling molecule can shoot up 1,000-fold or more during an acute illness. Focusing on low blood-plasma levels of CRP (less than 10 mg/L), Ridker demonstrated that healthy middle-aged men with extremely low levels—less than 0.5 mg/L—rarely have heart attacks,[6] while those men with levels greater than 3 mg/L have triple the risk of heart attack or stroke.[7-9] Furthermore, other studies show that the specificity of CRP in predicting a cardiovascular event is *extraordinarily* high.

The evidence reveals that CRP and other recognized clinical markers for inflammation (including fibrinogen and homocysteine) are strong predictive markers for a heart attack—far more predictive than the measure of cholesterol alone.[10-12] Several more studies propose that cholesterol may not pose any real danger at all, unless the fatty plaque is first weakened by the processes of inflammation and oxidative damage.[13;14]

Inflammation and Other Chronic Diseases

The more researchers probe systemic inflammation, the more they expose its links to other disease processes. Many researchers now believe that low-grade systemic inflammation is the basis for accelerated aging and the development of degenerative disease. Chronic inflammation is also an underlying cause of excess body fat and the inability to lose weight, and may be the important missing link in the current obesity epidemic.[15] It is associated with the onset of diabetes, Alzheimer's, Huntington's and Parkinson's diseases, amyotrophic lateral sclerosis, and multiple sclerosis, to name but a few. As well, several autoimmune diseases, such as rheumatoid arthritis, multiple sclerosis, lupus, and Crohn's disease can occur when there is too much *friendly fire* from the immune system.

The presence of activated microglial cells[*] in the brains of patients with neurodegenerative disorders is a strong clinical indicator of chronic inflammation in the central nervous system (CNS).[16] In a 25-year study evaluating the risks of dementia, men with high levels of CRP were up to three times more likely to contract Alzheimer's disease (AD) or vascular dementia than were men with low levels. Of note was the finding that silent, but deadly, inflammatory processes were evident long before clinical symptoms of dementia appeared.[17]

A recent study on inflammation and type 2 diabetes provides support for a common inflammatory basis for both AD and diabetes.[18] Diabetics have steeply elevated levels of inflammation, and many such individuals commonly suffer from both diseases. In patients with AD, inflammation of brain tissues increases the production of soluble beta-amyloid protein† and its conversion to insoluble amyloid fibrils. Accumulation of these harmful protein fibrils is closely associated with the deterioration of brain function. Moreover, because of a molecular structure that is similar to antibodies, the presence of beta-amyloid fibrils can overstimulate the immune system, leading to increased inflammation.[19;20] In type 2 diabetics, amyloid protein deposits similar to those found in the Alzheimer's brain can form in the pancreas, knocking out of action the cells responsible for the production of insulin. Chronically elevated levels of insulin and blood sugar, common to those suffering from metabolic syndrome (a prediabetic state characterized by increased insulin resistance and oxidative stress), trigger inflammatory events similar to those seen in AD that lead to the accumulation of these harmful protein plaques.

Chronic inflammation of the gastrointestinal tract can have far-reaching consequences, including the inability to absorb essential nutrients and the development of osteoporosis. Patients with inflammatory bowel disorder (IBD), a chronic inflammatory condition of the gut, demonstrate an inordinately high risk of osteoporosis.[21;22] Inflammation of the specialized cells lining the digestive tract appears to contribute to an imbalance in bone remodelling, triggering the release of bone destroying inflammatory proteins into the blood. This, in turn, leads to bone mineral loss and even greater systemic inflammation.[23]

> **Chronic inflammation is also an underlying cause of excess body fat and the inability to lose weight, and may be the important missing link in the current obesity epidemic.**

---

* *Microglial cells are the resident macrophages (specialized white blood cells) and the primary form of immune defence in the central nervous system (CNS). They scavenge damaged tissues, pump out harmful neurotoxins, and generate free radicals in response to inflammatory assaults.*

† *Amyloids are insoluble fibrous protein aggregations deposited in the brains of Alzheimer's patients. The name amyloid comes from the early mistaken identification of the substance as starch (amylum in Latin). It is not yet certain whether these fibrous plaques are a cause or a result of the disease.*

Inflammation also promotes several types of cancer. People with the highest blood levels of CRP and interleukin-6, another important inflammatory marker, are much more likely to contract colorectal, oesophageal, and other cancers than those with the lowest levels.[24-26] It is well known that nonsteroidal anti-inflammatory drugs (NSAIDs), such as aspirin and ibuprofen, reduce inflammation and with it the risk of contracting several types of cancer. [27;28]

Studies now show that systemic inflammation is involved in:

ALLERGY	HYPERTENSION
ALZHEIMER'S DISEASE	HEART ATTACK
ANEMIA	HUNTINGTON'S DISEASE
ANKYLOSING SPONDYLITIS	IRRITABLE BOWEL DISORDER
AORTIC VALVE STENOSIS	KIDNEY DISEASE
ARTHRITIS	LUPUS
CANCER	METABOLIC SYNDROME
CONGESTIVE HEART FAILURE	OSTEOPOROSIS
DIABETES	PARKINSON'S DISEASE
FIBROMYALGIA	PSORIASIS
FIBROSIS	STROKE

Inflammation, an indispensable survival mechanism from our evolutionary past, becomes our mortal enemy when it turns chronic. Understanding the process of chronic inflammation and learning how to tame its destructive forces is consequently critical to our long-term health.

What is Inflammation?

Viewed through its textbook definition, inflammation is a normal part of the body's defence against pathogens and injury. The increase in body temperature, the generation of toxic free radicals and inflammation-signalling molecules, and the release of specialized white blood cells (killer macrophages) are the hallmarks of an inflammatory event that is the body's means of defending against a clear and present danger. In modern man, however, this vigorous adaptive response, honed through millions of years of evolution, can become a harbinger of debilitating disease. The aging process may, in fact, be linked to the overexpression of the very defence mechanism that keeps us healthy when we are young.[29]

As we age, our ability to regulate inflammation diminishes. Then, rather than protecting us, inflammation morphs into a process of stealth through which degenerative disease can take root. The symptoms of chronic inflammation are entirely different from the cardinal signs of acute inflammation—*rubor* (redness), *calor* (heat), *tumor* (swelling), and *dolor* (pain)—and can lie undetected until calamity strikes.[19]

When inflammation turns silent, things get ugly. Silent inflammation is a chronic process that causes the body to turn on itself, its immune defences attacking its own organs.[30] Over time, dangerous inflammatory cytokines (specialized cell-signalling proteins) and inflammation-producing eicosanoids (oxygenated essential fatty acids) begin to destroy tissues throughout the body. In response to this attack from within, the body produces even more inflammatory agents and damaging free radicals, creating a self-perpetuating cycle of cellular damage.[31] Like a smouldering fire that slowly consumes itself, silent inflammation damages arteries, destroys nerve cells and organs, compromises the immune system, and promotes cancerous growths. If you have silent inflammation, despite how well you feel today, you may be on a fast track toward degenerative disease tomorrow.

The Inflammatory Cascade

Eicosanoids are a large class of fat-like molecules that are derived from the essential fatty acids, linoleic and alpha linolenic acid, supplied through our diet. Eicosanoids are actually primitive hormones from our evolutionary past; however, unlike the endocrine hormones that travel throughout the body, these specialized signalling molecules act only at the cellular level and only in the immediate vicinity where they are formed. The family of eicosanoids is large and includes several different classes: prostaglandins, thromboxanes, leukotrienes, lipoxins, isoprostanoids, endocannabinoids, and others.

These oxygenated fatty acids are the central players in the regulation of inflammation in the body; some eicosanoids are inflammatory, others are anti-inflammatory.

When inflammation turns silent, things get ugly. Silent inflammation is a chronic process that causes the body to turn on itself, its immune defences attacking its own organs.

Together, they form a command centre for the immune response, creating a dynamic balance between their opposing forces. When these forces get out of balance, systemic inflammation takes root.

Working in a coordinated fashion, eicosanoids can quickly shift the prevailing equilibrium to either *boost* or *dampen* the body's inflammatory response. The physiological effects of eicosanoids are far reaching: they are crucial to the regulation of blood pressure, blood clotting, heart and kidney function, allergic response, nerve transmission, hormone synthesis, and steroid production.

The Bad Eicosanoids

The inflammatory (*bad*) eicosanoids include several prostaglandins, which cause pain, and leukotrienes, which cause swelling. While certainly necessary in the body's defence against acute trauma and infection, their continued *over*expression is a significant factor in the onset of degenerative disease. Both classes of these inflammatory molecules are manufactured from arachidonic acid (AA), a fatty acid prevalent in red meats, shellfish, egg yolks, and other animal-based products. Arachidonic acid is manufactured in the body from conversion of linoleic acid, an *omega 6* essential fatty acid found in the oils extracted from several plant species, including poppy seed, safflower, sunflower, corn, and soybean oils. Evening primrose oil, black currant seed oil, and borage oil are also rich sources of linoleic acid.

Prostaglandin E2 (PG-E2) is a principal inflammatory eicosanoid. Release of this cell-signalling molecule will activate specialized white blood cells (macrophages) to search out and destroy invading pathogens. When released, PG-E2 promotes platelet stickiness, hardening of the arteries, heart attacks, and strokes.

PG-E2 will also activate the release of inflammatory cytokines, special signalling proteins that help coordinate the body's immune response.

Leukotriene B4 (LT-B4) another major inflammatory eicosanoid, is associated with several inflammatory conditions, including arthritis, asthma, atherosclerosis, and inflammatory bowel disease.[32-34] Likewise, thromboxane A2 (Tx-A2) is a powerful constrictor of vascular and respiratory smooth muscles. Excessive

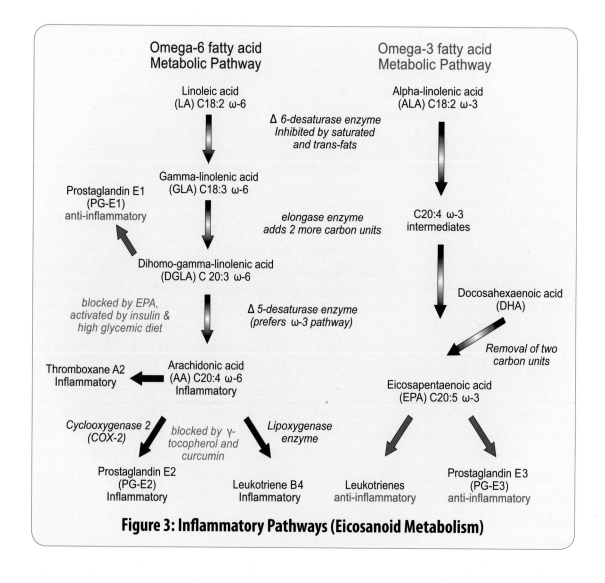

Figure 3: Inflammatory Pathways (Eicosanoid Metabolism)

production of Tx-A2 leads to high blood pressure.

The Good Eicosanoids

The good eicosanoids include prostaglandins E1 and E3 (PG-E1 and PG-E3) and several leukotrienes. They are manufactured from eicosapentaenoic acid (EPA). EPA is converted by the body from alpha linolenic acid (ALA), an *omega 3* essential fatty acid found in flax, canola, and pumpkin seeds. Flax seed is a particularly rich source of this protective essential fatty acid, containing up to 58% by weight of ALA. EPA is also found in the oils of fatty cold-water fish, including cod, mackerel, herring, salmon, and sardines. PG-E1 and PG-E3 are strongly anti-inflammatory; their production serves to dampen the immune response and return the body to a normal physiological state.

Docosahexaenoic acid (DHA), another important omega 3 fatty acid found in fish oils, is a major constituent of the fatty matrix in sperm, brain, and retinal tissues. DHA contributes to eicosanoid synthesis through its conversion by the body to EPA. Not only do EPA and DHA manufacture *good* eicosanoids, these indispensable omega 3 fats also inhibit the formation of inflammatory AA. This has the added benefit of reducing the downstream production of inflammatory (bad) eicosanoids.

Dietary supplementation with fish oil serves as a double whammy to the body's inflammatory response. First, fish oil ramps up the production of *good* eicosanoids by providing the needed substrates (EPA and DHA), which activate the protective omega 3 metabolic pathway. Second, fish oil blocks the production of the *bad* eicosanoids and hinders the formation of inflammation-promoting AA. Nutritional experts believe that daily consumption of high quality fish oil is *the single most important thing* you can do to tame the fires of chronic inflammation and reduce the risk of disease.

For further information on eicosanoid metabolism, please refer to Figure 3, opposite, which shows the two principal pathways responsible for modulating the body's inflammatory cascade.

Protecting Against Chronic Inflammation

When opposing *good* and *bad* eicosanoids are in balance, a state of wellness prevails; however, when they become chronically unbalanced problems arise. This balance is highly dependent on the level of insulin in the body.[38] High insulin levels—whether induced by chronic sugar overload, the onset of insulin resistance, or the hormonal effects of excess fat—set the stage for systemic inflammation. When insulin levels climb, oxidative assaults on the cell increase dramatically; in response, the cell mounts a protective defence, converting omega 6 fatty acids to inflammation-signalling molecules (prostaglandin E2, thromboxane A2, and leukotriene

B4). Chronically high blood insulin also increases the production of interleukin-6 (IL-6), another inflammatory cytokine that raises blood levels of CRP.

Apart from being far too high in refined sugar, the average North American diet is over-stuffed with inflammation-promoting omega 6 fats and scarce in inflammation-reducing omega 3 fats. This chronic fatty acid imbalance in the diet causes the body to bolster its inflammatory defences. As systemic inflammation rises, so does the production of cortisol, an antistress hormone that attempts to restore balance. Produced within the adrenal glands, cortisol is intricately involved in the body's response to stress. Problematically, in attempting to dampen inflammation, cortisol increases blood pressure, elevates blood-sugar levels, and suppresses the immune system. Chronically elevated cortisol also places physiological stress on all organs and increases the risk of degenerative disease.

Researchers contend that the stimulatory effects of high insulin levels, overconsumption of high-glycemic foods, and chronic deficiency in healthy omega 3 fatty acids, typical of our modern diet, *directly* implicate diet and obesity in the damage caused by chronic inflammation.

Fortunately, changing the balance within the body to favour the production of anti-inflammatory messengers is surprisingly easy: simply increase your daily intake of inflammation-busting omega 3 fats and reduce your intake of inflammation-promoting omega 6 fats. Even eating a handful of fresh almonds, a rich source of inflammation-dampening gamma tocopherol (a form of vitamin E), reduces inflammation to about the same level as taking a first generation statin drug.[39]

When insulin levels are reduced through weight loss and dietary modification, production of anti-inflammatory prostaglandins is favoured and inflammation is kept in check.[40] The basic goal is to reduce the production and dietary intake of AA and increase the levels of healthy fats to promote the production of *good* prostaglandins.[41;42] The modern diet contains 10 to 20 times the amount of omega 6 oils that we need. Consequently, the most sensible dietary approach is to eliminate sources of omega 6 oils and supplement with high-dose omega 3 oils to return us to an optimal 4:1 ratio of omega 6 and omega 3 fatty acids.[43]

Decreasing your dietary intake of red meats, eggs, dairy, high-glycemic foods, and foods high in saturated fats will help reduce cellular levels of inflammation-promoting AA and shift the omega 6/omega 3 balance in favour of the beneficial omega 3 fats. As well, increasing your dietary intake of fatty fish, raw nuts and grains rich in healthy fats, and supplementing with a high quality cold-pressed fish oil or flaxseed oil will provide a safe, effective, and

> Overconsumption of high-glycemic foods, typical of our modern diet, *directly* implicate diet and obesity in the damage caused by chronic inflammation.

drug-free way to reduce your level of systemic inflammation—and with it your risk of degenerative disease.

Triggering the Inflammatory Cascade

Reducing insulin levels, cutting the intake of refined sugars, and optimizing the ratio of essential fatty acids will dampen systemic inflammation. However, these are not the only control mechanisms available to us.

It is well established that oxidative stress directly induces an inflammatory response by the cell.[44-47] Consequently, the answer to controlling *both* oxidative stress and inflammation lies in understanding the biochemical link between these two processes. Researchers have now identified a key signalling molecule that senses oxidative insults to the cell from external agents and swings into action to protect the cell.

Here is how it appears to unfold: oxidative assaults on the cell membrane from external stressors (infectious agents, high-glycemic foods, environmental toxins, etc.) causes lipid peroxidation* and the concurrent production of arachidonic acid (AA) within the membrane.[48] Next, AA is modified by enzymes, yielding several inflammation-promoting agents that migrate into the cytoplasm of the cell. This triggers an initial inflammatory response from the cell. In self-defence, free radical production *within* the cell is amplified. This, in turn, activates an important nuclear transcription molecule called nuclear factor kappa beta (NF-kB).

The Link to Oxidative Stress

As a first responder within the cell, NF-kB acts much like a smoke detector, monitoring the cell's internal environment for early signs of danger. Present in the cytoplasm of the cell, NF-kB is normally bound to a protein that keeps it in an inactive state. Once activated, this critically important cell-signalling molecule migrates to the nucleus of the cell, attaching to specific sites along the DNA (the cell's genetic blueprint). Here it commands the transcription (copying) of over 400 genes that control the manufacture of numerous inflammation-promoting molecules.[49] Once manufactured in the cytoplasm of the cell, these chemical 'foot soldiers' immediately ramp up the cell's inflammatory response against the invader.

> So we see that because of the actions of NF-kB, oxidative stress promotes inflammation and, conversely, inflammation promotes oxidative stress.

---

* *Lipid peroxidation is the autocatalytic oxidative degradation of lipids that proceeds through a free-radical chain reaction mechanism. Left unchecked, lipid peroxidation causes extensive damage to the integrity of membrane structures of the cell.*

As the master switch for inflammation, NF-kB controls the genes encoding a diverse range of signalling molecules, all of them central to the inflammatory cascade and all of them capable of augmenting the level of oxidative stress. So we see that, because of the actions of NF-kB, oxidative stress promotes inflammation and, conversely, inflammation promotes oxidative stress.

> Simply put, we have to stop digging our graves with our own knife and fork.

For several years, Life Extension Foundation (LEF), a Florida-based research organization dedicated to exploring aging and chronic disease, has been warning about the dangers of overexpression of NF-kB. Through their work, we now know that expression of NF-kB in the body increases as we age, provoking systemic inflammation and setting the stage for the progression of degenerative disease.[49] Inflammation is now thought to be the initiating factor in most degenerative diseases and is estimated to underlie up to 98% of all diseases afflicting humans.[50]

Nature to the Rescue

Fortunately, nature has provided generously for our protection with plant-based nutrients that can help dampen the overexpression of NF-kB. The polyphenols, with well over 8,000 known structural variants, are the most prolific family of NF-kB inhibitors known to science. Polyphenols are secondary metabolites of plants—effective free radical antagonists and metal chelators that comprise a vast range of complex molecular structures. Polyphenols include several constituents found in olive oil; the citrus bioflavonoids, found in fruits and berries; resveratrol, found in red wine and grapes; curcumin, isolated from turmeric (*Curcuma longa*) rhizome; and the catechins, isolated from green tea, grape seeds, assorted nuts and berries, and pine bark. The remarkable health-protective benefits of the Mediterranean diet are largely attributed to the quantities of polyphenols found in the food groups consumed in this diet.

While early research on polyphenols viewed these substances as antioxidants, later studies showed that polyphenols effectively regulate cellular processes that control inflammatory events and may, themselves, serve as signalling agents to temper inflammation.[51] The capacity of polyphenols to inhibit NF-kB is absolutely critical to the ability of the cell to reduce inflammation; this is why a diet high in fresh fruits and vegetables is so important to long-term health.[52]

Many other natural compounds exert beneficial effects through interaction with NF-kB. Early investigations showed that supplementation with alpha lipoic acid (ALA), an important antioxidant found in higher quality nutritional supplements, can stimulate the production of anti-inflammatory prostaglandins.[53] ALA has also been found to bind to and inhibit NF-kB within the cell's nucleus[54] and can act as a therapeutic agent against bone loss associated with systemic inflammation of the gut. Present in both the lipid and aqueous phases of the cell, ALA can also penetrate the blood-brain barrier with ease to protect the central nervous system from inflammatory events.

While most antioxidants demonstrate some level of anti-inflammatory activity, vitamin C, in particular, reduces blood levels of several inflammatory markers, including the inflammatory proteins associated with NF-kB activation.[58-60] As well, n-acetyl cysteine and s-adenosyl methionine are strong inhibitors of NF-kB.[61] So too, the fatty acids EPA and DHA found in fish oil, apart from their ability to impede the inflammatory AA pathway, directly inhibit NF-kB activity.

Implications

Systemic, low-grade, chronic inflammation is an underlying cause of the vast majority of degenerative diseases that are the principal causes of nonaccidental death in today's world. The fact that this type of inflammation increases with age and with poor dietary and lifestyle choices means that most people unknowingly suffer from this silent, but deadly, disorder.

Yet, it does not have to be like this. We have the solution at hand to resolve this dilemma: all that is necessary is to understand that what we put *into* our bodies and what we do *with* our bodies will largely determine our longevity and quality of life. Cutting down today on unnecessary exposure to environmental toxins and those elements in our diet that promote inflammation will decidedly reduce our risk of dying tomorrow from cancer or cardiovascular disease.

Simply put, we have to stop digging our graves with our own knife and fork—it all comes down to the choices we make along the way.

Nations endure only as long as their topsoil.

~Henry Cantwell Wallace (1866 - 1924)
US Secretary of Agriculture from 1921-1924

CHAPTER THREE:

NUTRIENT DEPLETION OF OUR FOODS

We are made of the stuff of the earth.

Our daily bread comes from the plants that form the roots of the human food chain. They provide us with important macronutrients, the carbohydrates, proteins, fats, and oils that are manufactured through photosynthesis and are needed to fuel our bodies. Plants also provide us with important micronutrients, the vitamins manufactured by the plant and the minerals absorbed from the soils, which are obligatory for healthy cellular function.

Vitamins and minerals serve as essential components in enzymes and coenzymes (helper enzymes), the biological catalysts that speed up chemical reactions necessary for cellular function. They work in concert to either join molecules together or break them apart in countless chemical reactions that take place every second within the living cell. Simply put, without enzymes and their essential vitamins and minerals, life could not exist.

Reflecting on this, the calculus becomes simple: plants can't make minerals; they must absorb them from the soil—and without minerals, vitamins don't work. Accordingly, if important minerals are depleted from our soils, they are *also* depleted from our bodies.

This we also know: chronic mineral deficiency leads to disease. Consequently, it is not surprising that any degradation in the nutrient content of our soils leads to a commensurate increase in nutritionally related diseases in both animal and human populations.

The bottom line is that our physical health ultimately depends upon the health of our topsoil.

The alarming fact is that foods—fruits, vegetables and grains—now being raised on millions of acres of land that no longer contain enough of certain needed nutrients, are starving us—no matter how much we eat of them.
~US Senate Document 264

The remarkable thing about the above declaration, found in US Senate document

264, is that it was issued *nearly eight decades* ago in 1936. Since that time, the United States and other industrialized nations have been losing arable land at an unprecedented rate. In the United States topsoil is eroding at a rate today that is ten times greater than the rate of replenishment. In countries such as Africa, India, and China soil erosion exceeds the replenishment rate by 30 to 40 times. Current estimates place the chronological reserves of our global topsoil at less than 50 years. As the topsoil goes, so go the vital nutrients—and so goes our health.[1]

Findings released at the 1992 RIO Earth Summit confirmed that mineral depletion of our global topsoil reserve was rampant throughout the 20th century. During that time, US and Canadian agricultural soils lost 85% of their mineral content; Asian and South American soils dropped 76%; and throughout Africa, Europe, and Australia soil mineral content was depleted by 72-74%.[1] The Rio summit concluded: "There is deep concern over continuing major declines in the mineral values in farm and range soils throughout the world." That was almost a quarter century ago and little has been done since to forestall the inevitable exhaustion of these precious mineral stores.

In March, 2006 the United Nations recognized a new kind of malnutrition: *multiple micronutrient depletion*. According to Catherine Bertini, Chair of the UN Standing Committee on Nutrition, the overweight are *just* as malnourished as the starving. In essence, it is not the *quantity* of food that is at issue—it is the *quality*.[2]

Modern Agriculture Impoverishes our Soils

The earth's topsoils are a wafer-thin envelope of mineral-containing, carbon-based materials. Soils act to buffer and filter water and airborne pollutants, store critical moisture and important minerals and micronutrients, and are essential reservoirs for carbon dioxide and methane. Global warming aside, soil degradation is one of the most ominous threats to the long-term environmental sustainability of our planet.

Soil depletion was well understood in primitive societies, which would migrate every few years to new lands or would replenish the soils with organic wastes. In more recent history, the western migration of Europeans to the New World witnessed families moving every few years as their dryland farming practices repeatedly played out the soil. The first sign of nutrient exhaustion did not come from crop failure; rather, it appeared as increased illness and disease amongst both the animals and humans who relied upon the land.[3] Those who did not leave their farms observed inevitable declines in crop production, followed by outright collapse of the land, as was witnessed in the great dust bowl formations throughout the American mid west during the 1930s.

Today, we have nowhere else to go. We can no longer simply pick up and leave for greener pastures because there are none left. We must make do with what we have—soil erosion, contamination with industrial pollutants, and depletion of our limited mineral resources have now gone global.[4-11] Nevertheless, modern agricultural practices continue to consume water, fuel, and topsoil at alarmingly unsustainable rates, seemingly oblivious to nature's inviolate dictate to give back to the earth what we have taken. Instead of renewing and replenishing our soils, commercial agriculture has corrupted nature's cycles, and for this there will be a steep price to pay.

> The US Department of Agriculture standards for fruits and vegetables are limited to size, shape, and colour—they do not even consider nutritional value.

Impoverished Soils, Impoverished Crops

Soil depletion through unsustainable agricultural practices results in an inevitable loss of nutrient content in our crops. Data compiled by the US-based Nutrition Security Institute, clearly demonstrate the precipitous drop in the nutrient content of selected produce over the last century.[1] As shown in the following graph, between 1914 and 1997 the summed average content of calcium, magnesium, and iron in cabbage, tomatoes, and spinach fell from 400 milligrams to about 75 milligrams.

Later research published in the *Journal of the American College of Nutrition* in

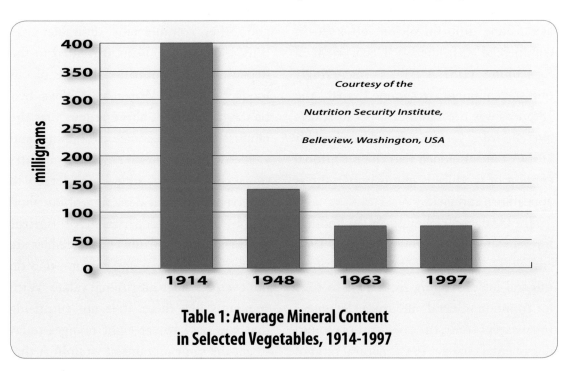

Courtesy of the

Nutrition Security Institute,

Belleview, Washington, USA

Table 1: Average Mineral Content in Selected Vegetables, 1914-1997

2004 confirms continued declines in the content of several nutrients amongst 43 garden crops grown in US markets from 1950 to 1999.[12]

A 2001 investigative report published by Florida-based Life Extension Foundation reveals that the vitamin and mineral content of several foods dropped dramatically between 1963 and 2000. Collard greens showed a 62% loss of vitamin C, a 41% loss of vitamin A, and a 29% loss of calcium. Similarly, potassium and magnesium were down 52% and 84%. Cauliflower had lost almost half of its vitamin C, thiamine, and riboflavin, and most of the calcium in commercial pineapples had all but disappeared. When asked to explain the astonishing drop in calcium observed in commercial corn, the US Department of Agriculture (USDA), in a staggeringly obtuse comment, responded that the 78% loss was not significant because, *"No one eats corn for calcium."* Unbelievably, USDA officials added that the nutritional content of produce is not as important as appearance and yield.[13]

The US data corroborate similar findings for vegetable crops grown between 1940 and 2002 in Great Britain, which show mineral losses ranging from 15% to 62% for common minerals and trace elements.[2] In an earlier study, the same authors found detrimental changes in the natural ratio of

> Pesticides and herbicides have been linked to a wide range of human health effects, including immune suppression, hormone disruption, diminished intelligence, reproductive abnormalities, neurological and behavioral disorders, and cancer.

minerals, such as calcium and magnesium, in the foods tested.[14] Similarly, a Canadian study found dramatic declines in the nutrient content of produce grown over a 50 year interval to 1999. During that time the average Canadian spud lost 57% of its vitamin C and iron, 28% of its calcium, 50% of its riboflavin, and 18% of its niacin. The story was the same for all 25 fruits and vegetables analyzed. The Canadian data revealed that nearly 80% of the foods tested showed large drops in their calcium and iron content, three fourths showed significant decreases in vitamin A, one half lost vitamin C and riboflavin, and one third lost thiamine.[15]

Selective breeding of new crop varieties that places a premium on yield, appearance, and other commercially desirable characteristics has also been attributed to the depletion of the nutritional value of our foods.[16] Dr Phil Warman of Nova Scotia's Agricultural College argues that the emphasis on appearance, storability, and yield—with little or no emphasis on nutritional content—has added considerably to the overall nutrient depletion of our food supply. The US Department of Agriculture standards for fruits and vegetables are limited to size, shape, and colour—they do not even consider nutritional value.[1] With standards like these, it is not surprising that you have to eat eight oranges today to get the same amount of vitamin A that your grandparents got from a *single* orange.[15]

A 2006 British study shows that, as would be expected, mineral losses in animal products reflect those in plant foods. Comparing levels measured in 2002 with those present in 1940, the iron content of milk was found to be 62% less, calcium and magnesium in Parmesan cheese had each fallen by 70%, and copper in dairy produce had plummeted by a remarkable 90%.[17]

How Nutrients are Removed from Soils

Erosion of topsoil by wind and water is accelerated by overcultivating, overgrazing, and destruction of natural ground cover. The loss of organic matter results in a concurrent loss of nitrogen, minerals, and trace elements. It also reduces the ability of soil to hold moisture and support the growth of healthy plants. The nutrient demands from high-yield crops place a further burden on the limited nutritional capacity of already depleted soils. For example, in 1930 an acre of land would yield about 50 bushels of corn. By 1960, yields had reached 200 bushels per acre, far beyond the capacity of the soil to sustain itself.[18]

Erosion, in combination with high-yield nutrient extraction, also depletes the soil of its alkalizing minerals (calcium, potassium, and magnesium). This loss of natural buffering capacity results in the release of acids from natural clay deposits, causing the soil to become increasingly acidic. Conversely, overirrigation with hard water causes some soils to leach important minerals while accumulating others (such as calcium and magnesium). As a result, the soil becomes too alkaline to sustain crop growth.

Nitrate, phosphate, and potassium (NPK) fertilizers, first introduced in the early 1900s, significantly increase crop yield, but they do so at great expense. Overuse of these chemical fertilizers has been found to *accelerate* the depletion of other vital micronutrients and trace elements and reduce their bioavailability to plants.[19] NPK fertilizers will gradually reduce soil pH,* rendering the soils too acidic to support beneficial bacteria and fungi. These important symbiotic organisms assist the plant in absorbing nutrients from the soil. Once gone, uptake of micronutrients by plants is significantly impaired.[20] Moreover, in acidic soils, NPK application has been found to bind soil-based selenium, making it unavailable for root absorption.[21]

The use of NPK fertilizers to replenish the principal growth-promoting nutrients fails to address the concurrent losses of valuable micronutrients and trace elements (such as copper, zinc, and molybdenum) which occur in intensively cultivated soils.

---

* *pH (power of hydrogen) is a chemical term that represents the level of acidity based on the molar concentration of hydrogen ions in solution.*

According to Dr William Albrecht of the University of Missouri, the use of NPK fertilizers ultimately leads to malnutrition; attack by insects, bacteria, and fungi; weed encroachment; and crop loss in dry weather.[22] Albrecht contends that the use of chemical fertilizers to chase yield actually *weakens* the crop, making it *more* susceptible to pests and disease. Consequently, the commercial farmer has no choice but to rely on harmful chemical pesticides to protect his crop and his investment.

> No matter how conscientious we may be, we are constantly exposed—through the foods we eat, the water we drink, and the air we breathe—to environmental levels of these toxins.

Nutrient Depletion forces Pesticide Abuse

The weakening of both soils and crops through the indiscriminate practices of commercial agriculture creates an overwhelming dependence on the use of pesticides and herbicides in order to maintain crop yield. These toxic organochloride (OC) and organophosphate (OP) compounds kill our soils by slaughtering the symbiotic bacteria and fungi that promote nutrient uptake in plants. They also inactivate critical enzyme systems within the plant roots that are involved in mineral absorption,[20] and they destroy the soil micro-organisms needed to create the organic/mineral complexes that naturally replenish the soil.[19]

To make matters worse, these environmental poisons end up on our dinner table.

Dr Jerome Weisner, Science Advisor for President John F Kennedy, said in 1963: "The use of pesticides is far more dangerous than radioactive fallout." Unfortunately, he may have underestimated their potential for harm. Most atmospheric radioactive fallout soon decays to harmless background levels. Pesticides, on the other hand, are *persistent* environmental toxins that accumulate and concentrate along the food chain, their residues sequestered in the fatty tissues of the body. All of us carry a lifetime body burden of these environmental poisons and many of us unknowingly suffer their cumulative effects.

Human exposure to pesticides is pervasive and occurs most commonly through the food we eat.[23-47] While some studies have attempted to refute the claim that exposure to pesticide residues is detrimental,[48-50] there is a great body of evidence that pesticides can elicit harmful biological effects—sometimes at exquisitely low levels[25;26;44;51]—as a result of chronic exposure.[27;38;52;53]

Moreover, dangerous synergistic effects from combinations of pesticides and chemical agents can occur at normal levels of environmental exposure.[38;54] In some studies, pesticide cocktails have been found to elicit toxic effects at levels significantly *below* those expressed by the individual chemicals.[55-58] In one investigation, a cocktail of aldicarb, atrazine, and nitrate, at levels approximate to those found in groundwater across the United States, induced endocrine, immune, and behavioral changes at doses that—for the individual compounds at the same concentrations—could not be observed.[57]

While the industry continues to claim that pesticides and herbicides are safe and effective, a recent study suggests that women with breast cancer are five to nine times more likely to have significant levels of pesticide residues in their blood.[59] As well, pesticides and herbicides have been linked to a wide range of human health effects, including immune suppression, hormone disruption, diminished intelligence, reproductive abnormalities, neurological and behavioral disorders, and cancer.[52;53] They are also potent endocrine hormone disruptors and can be passed easily through the placenta to the unborn infant, who is extremely vulnerable to toxins that disrupt the developmental process.[60-63] Children are particularly susceptible to pesticides because of a higher level of food intake for their body weight and a still-maturing immune system.

To increase resistance to pesticides and herbicides in commercially grown crops and maximize yield, the agro-food industry has now turned to the use of genetically modified organisms. While no systematic or clinical studies on the safety of genetically modified (GMO) foods currently exist, adverse microscopic and molecular effects in different organs and tissues have been reported.[64] Some investigations reveal evidence of harm from the consumption of such foods, although the mechanism remains to be explained.[65] The results of most studies indicate that GMO foods may cause hepatic, pancreatic, renal, or reproductive effects and may alter blood chemistry and impact the body's immune system.[66] Because genetic modification techniques alter specific proteins expressed by the plant, it is understandable that certain GMO foods can elicit harmful allergic responses in sensitive individuals.[67-69]

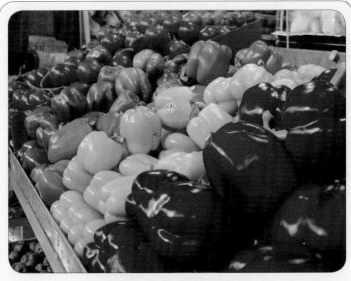

Figure 4: Healthy Foods
Organically grown fruits and vegetables have much higher levels of vitamins, minerals, and antioxidants, and much lower levels of pesticide contaminants, than factory-farmed produce.

Shockingly, over 300 food additives, including aspartame, phosphoric acid, monosodium glutamate, transhydrogenated fats and various preservatives, stabilizers, artificial sweeteners and colourings, are allowed in conventional foods. Food colourings have been shown to have a wide range of harmful effects. Tartrazine (Yellow E102), for example, has been linked to severe allergic response, headaches, asthma, growth retardation, and hyperactivity disorder in children.[70;71] Artificial sweeteners, colourings, and most chemical additives are *banned* in certified organically grown foods.

No matter how conscientious we may be, we are constantly exposed—through the foods we eat, the water we drink, and the air we breathe—to environmental levels of these toxins that may manifest in subtle or profound ways. For this reason, it is exceedingly important to protect yourself and your children, as much as you can, by choosing sensible dietary alternatives to commercially gown and processed foods, the principal sources of pesticide exposure.

> The fact is, unless we supplement, most of us do not even come close to meeting our daily nutritional requirements for vitamins, minerals, and trace elements.

Organic Agriculture Improves Nutrient Content

For most of human history, agriculture has used organic growing practices. Only during the last 100 years has the use of synthetic chemicals and their widely destructive consequences been introduced to the food supply. Fortunately, an increasing number of progressive growers are, today, shunning commercial growing techniques; instead, they are returning to their organic roots and the traditional ways of caring for the soil.

The natural mulching and cultivation techniques employed through organic gardening feed the soil rather than the plant by returning many of the nutrients lost through plant growth and by encouraging the growth of fungi, nitrogen-fixing bacteria, and other beneficial micro-organisms. Healthy *living* soil, in turn, promotes the symbiosis of plants with these soil microbes, thereby enhancing the transfer of essential nutrients into the plants. In contrast to conventional agriculture, organic agriculture *embraces* the natural replenishing cycles of nature.

In a 2003 exposure study in Seattle, Washington, children two-to-four years of age who consumed organically grown fruits and vegetables had urine levels of pesticides six times lower than children who consumed conventionally grown foods. According to the authors of the study, the consumption of organic fruits, vegetables, and juices can reduce children's exposure levels from *above* to *below* the US Environmental Protection Agency's current guidelines, thereby shifting exposures from a range of *uncertain* risk to a range of *negligible* risk.[72]

There is a growing body of evidence confirming the health-promoting effects of organically grown foods. Studies confirm that organic crops are higher in vitamin C, iron, natural sugars, magnesium, phosphorus, and other minerals, and lower in harmful nitrates than are conventional crops.[73;74] An independent review, published in the *Journal of Complementary Medicine*, found that organic crops had markedly higher levels of all 21 nutrients evaluated in the study than did conventionally grown produce. Organically grown spinach, lettuce, cabbage, and potatoes expressed particularly high levels of minerals.[74]

Research conducted by the University of California, Davis, showed that organically grown tomatoes and peppers had higher levels of flavonoids* and vitamin C than conventionally grown tomatoes.[75] The health-promoting effects of these secondary plant metabolites, manufactured by the plant to protect it from the oxidative damage caused by strong sunlight, are well established. High intensity conventional agricultural practices appear to disrupt the natural production of these plant metabolites, leading to a loss of flavonoid content in conventional crops. Conversely, organic growing practices are known to stimulate the plant's defence mechanisms, leading to enhanced production of these important plant-based nutrients.[76] It

is precisely because organic crops are not protected by pesticides that their fruits contain higher levels of flavonoids than conventional fruits—including up to 50% more antioxidants.[76-78] A good example is the polyphenol content of red wine. This heart-healthy nutrient is found in much higher concentrations in wine made from organically grown grapes, which manufacture the nutrient to protect against a naturally occurring fungus that can attack the skin of the grape.

Conclusions

The conveniences of modern living involve many compromises when it comes to eating a healthy diet. Most of us are completely unaware of the consequences of chronic exposure to persistent environmental toxins through the chemically laced foods we regularly place on our dinner table. Nor do we appreciate the degree to which the nutritional value of our food supply has been bludgeoned by our over-reliance on commercial, chemically based agriculture. The fact is, unless we supplement, most of us do not even come close to meeting our daily nutritional requirements for vitamins, minerals, and trace elements. Less than one third of us eat the recommended servings of fruits and vegetables every day.

---

* *Flavonoids are a group of plant pigments that are responsible for the bright colours of many fruits and flowers. Designed by nature to protect the plant against the damage caused by sun exposure and disease, they elicit powerful antioxidant, cell signalling, and anti-inflammatory properties.*

Now we find that even if a person accidentally *does* eat a vegetable, it doesn't have nearly the nutrition that nature intended.

What Choices Do We Have?

To start with, we can begin to identify those foods most highly exposed to chemical fertilizers and choose to complement our diets with organically grown alternatives. We can learn how to grow our own produce on family-owned or community garden plots and use organic growing techniques, such as composting and feeding the soil, to replenish the nutrients. If we can't grow our own gardens, we can choose to support local farmers and agriculturalists, encouraging the growth of a local organic farming culture, and we can support organic growers the world over with the purchase power of our consumer dollar. Within the home, we can learn to adapt culinary and cooking techniques, such as steaming and stir

> Now we find that even if a person accidentally *does* eat a vegetable, it doesn't have nearly the nutrition that nature intended.

frying that *optimize*, rather than *compromise,* the nutritional value of the foods we purchase. We can also learn to stop treating vegetables as a *side* dish and prepare our meals with the understanding that optimal nutritional intake of fresh fruits and vegetables is our best defense against illness and disease.

Finally, we must accept the fact that, despite our best intentions to eat a balanced diet, the dictates of modern lifestyles and prevalence of ready-made meals that now pervade the culture throughout the Americas make it extraordinarily difficult to do so. That is why daily supplementation with a high quality, broad-spectrum nutritional supplement—one with a full range of the necessary vitamins, minerals, and plant-based antioxidants—is a prudent preventive measure to reduce the risk of chronic disease and promote long-term health.

And that is precisely what the venerated American Medical Association now recommends.

> **Vitamins, if properly understood and applied, will help us to reduce human suffering to an extent which the most fantastic human mind would fail to imagine.**
>
> ~ *Albert Szent-Györgyi (1893–1986)*
> *Nobel Laureate, Physiology and Medicine*

CHAPTER FOUR:

WHY WE NEED TO SUPPLEMENT

The word is out: it pays to take your vitamins.

In 2002, the American Medical Association (AMA) reversed its long-held antivitamin stance and began to encourage all adults to supplement daily with a multiple vitamin. A landmark review of 38 years of scientific evidence by Harvard researchers Drs Robert Fletcher and Kathleen Fairfield convinced the conservative *Journal of the American Medical Association (JAMA)* to rewrite its policy guidelines regarding the use of vitamin supplements. In two reports, published in the June 19, 2002 edition of *JAMA,* the authors concluded that the current North American diet, while sufficient to prevent acute vitamin deficiency diseases, such as scurvy and pellagra, is inadequate to support long-term health.[1;2]

Insufficient vitamin intake is apparently a cause of chronic diseases. Recent evidence has shown that suboptimal levels of vitamins (below standard), even well above those causing deficiency syndromes, are risk factors for chronic diseases such as cardiovascular disease, cancer, and osteoporosis. A large portion of the general population is apparently at increased risk for this reason.

~ **Drs Robert Fletcher and Kathleen Fairfield**

In the study the authors examined several nutrients, including vitamins A, B_6, B_{12}, C, D, E, K, folic acid, and several of the carotenoids (including alpha- and beta carotene, cryptoxanthin, zeaxanthin, lycopene, and lutein). Among their conclusions, they noted:

✓ folic acid, vitamin B_6, and vitamin B_{12} are required for proper homocysteine metabolism and low levels of these vitamins are associated with increased risk of heart disease (homocysteine is a sulfur-containing amino acid that, at high blood levels, can damage the cardiovascular system);

✓ inadequate folic acid status increases the risk of neural tube defects and some cancers (a neural tube defect is an incomplete closing of the spinal cord that occurs early in foetal development);

✓ vitamin E and lycopene (the red pigment found in ripe tomatoes) appear to decrease the risk of prostate cancer;

✓ vitamin D is associated with a decreased risk of osteoporosis and fracture when taken with calcium (osteoporosis is a hollowing out of the of the bones, caused by the loss of calcium);

✓ inadequate vitamin B_{12} is associated with anaemia and neurological disorders (anaemia is a decrease in number of red blood cells or a lack of hemoglobin in the blood);

✓ low dietary levels of carotenoids, the brightly coloured pigments in peppers, carrots, and fruits, appear to increase the risk of breast, prostate, and lung cancers (carotenoids belong to the family of nutrients called bioflavonoids);

✓ inadequate vitamin C is associated with increased cancer risk; and

✓ low levels of vitamin A are associated with vision disorders and impaired immune function.

In a striking departure from *JAMA's* previous antivitamin stance, the authors concluded that, given our modern diet, supplementation each day with a multiple vitamin is a prudent preventive measure against chronic disease. The researchers based their guidance on the fact that more than 80% of the American population does not consume anywhere near the five servings of fruits and vegetables required each day for optimal health.

JAMA's previous comprehensive review of vitamins, conducted in the 1980s, concluded that people of normal health do not need to take a multivitamin and can meet all their nutritional needs through diet alone. Since that time, nutritional science has compiled an impressive wealth of studies affirming the health benefits of supplementation as an adjunct to a healthy diet. The American Medical Association's about-face, in light of the Fairfield/Fletcher studies, and its public declaration that supplementation is now deemed important to your health, underscores the strength of the scientific evidence that now prevails.

The Case for Supplementation

We now have convincing evidence that the lifetime risk of cancer; heart disease; stroke; diabetes; neurological disorders, such as multiple sclerosis and amyotrophic lateral sclerosis (Lou Gehrig's disease); macular degeneration; osteoporosis; Alzheimer's disease; and other forms of dementia can be reduced by providing the cells of the body with sufficient amounts of the right nutrients.

One of the first human studies to substantiate the benefits of vitamin supplements was announced in 1992 and showed that men who took 800 mg/day of vitamin C lived six years longer than those who consumed the US Food and Nutrition Board's recommended daily allowance of 60 mg/day.[3]

Published in the journal *Epidemiology*, this ten year followup study showed that high vitamin C intake extended average life span and reduced mortality from both cardiovascular disease and cancer.[4]

A compelling report that higher potency supplements extend human life span was published in August, 1996 in the *American Journal of Clinical Nutrition*. The study involved 11,178 elderly people who participated in a trial to establish the effects of vitamin supplements on mortality. Supplementation with vitamin E alone reduced the risk of overall mortality by 34% and reduced the risk of coronary disease mortality by 47%. However, when vitamin C and E were used in combination, overall mortality was reduced by 42% and coronary mortality dropped by 53%, demonstrating the synergistic effects of multiple vitamin therapy. What made these findings of even greater significance was that the study compared people who took low-potency one-a-day multiple vitamins to those who took higher potency vitamin C and E supplements. Only those participants taking high-dose vitamin C and E supplements benefitted.[3;5]

A 1997 study published in the *British Medical Journal* evaluated 1,605 healthy men with no evidence of pre-existing heart disease. Those men deficient in vitamin C were found to have a 350% increased incidence of sudden heart attacks compared to those who were not deficient in vitamin C. The authors concluded that vitamin C deficiency, as measured by low blood levels of ascorbate, is a significant risk factor for coronary heart disease.[6]

A massive cohort study, published in 1998, investigated the risk for colon cancer in 88,756 nurses who took folic acid (a B-complex vitamin) as part of a daily multivitamin supplement.[7] The study found that intakes of 400 mg/day or more of folate, compared to intakes of 200 mg/day or less, were strongly related to lowered risk. While no significant protective effects were noted over shorter periods, an inverse relationship between folate intake and cancer risk became apparent after five years of use. After 15 years, a remarkable 75% reduction in the risk of colon cancer was noted among those women taking the supplements containing the B-complex vitamin. The authors concluded that long-term use of multivitamins might substantially reduce the risk for colon cancer, an effect likely related to the folic acid contained in these products.

In this same study, nurses who took multivitamins containing vitamin B_6 also reduced their risk of heart attack by 30%. The evidence revealed that the more

> The authors concluded that, given our modern diet, supplementation each day with a multiple vitamin is a prudent preventive measure against chronic disease.

vitamin B_6 they took, the lower was the risk of suffering a sudden cardiac event. These findings support those of another cohort study conducted in Norway that demonstrated a combination of folic acid and vitamin B_6 can reduce homocysteine levels by up to 32% in healthy individuals. Homocysteine, a harmful amino acid at high blood levels, can markedly increase the level of inflammation and oxidative stress in blood vessels, which can precipitate both heart attack and stroke.[8]

In 2005, an international coalition led by Canadian researchers at McMaster University, Ontario provided evidence that a comprehensive cocktail of nutritional supplements can significantly improve lifespan in animal models. The nutrient mixture, containing 31 nutrients common to many better quality broad-spectrum supplements available in the market, targeted key factors in the aging process, including the proliferation of reactive oxygen species, inflammatory processes, insulin resistance, and mitochondrial* dysfunction. In the study, the treatment group of mice exhibited an 11% increase in lifespan compared to normal mice who did not receive the supplement cocktail. Previously, the same researchers showed that the supplement cocktail completely abolished severe cognitive decline expressed by aging untreated mice. The results from these animal-model experiments demonstrate that broad-spectrum dietary supplements may be effective in ameliorating the effects of aging and age-related pathologies where simpler formulations have generally failed.[9;10]

The benefits of supplementation with n-3 polyunsaturated fatty

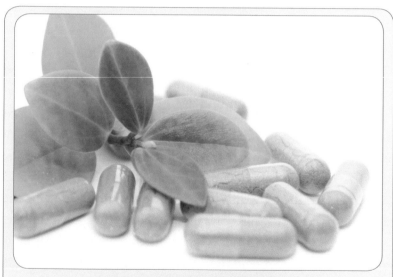

Figure 5: Dietary Supplements
We can help replace the nutrients missing from our diets with vitamins, minerals, and other micronutrients from supplements.

---

*   *Mitochondria are tiny organelles that are the power centres of the cell. It is in the mitochondria that many of the energy-producing reactions of cellular respiration take place. In the terminal process of respiration, reactive oxygen species are created that can damage the delicate membranes of these organelles if left unprotected through lack of antioxidants. Oxidative damage to the delicate mitochondrial membrane is believed to be a principal cause of cellular aging.*

acids (omega 3 fats) after a heart attack are well documented. Omega 3 fatty acids, commonly found in cold-water fish, nuts, and grains, dramatically reduce the risk of premature death in high risk individuals. A 2008 study on postmyocardial infarction (heart attack) patients revealed a significantly lower likelihood of dangerous cardiac arrhythmia and an 85% reduction in the risk of premature death

> These studies and their findings are but a few of the thousands of independent scientific studies supporting the value of supplementation with higher quality nutritional supplements.

by simply maintaining an optimal level of omega 3 fats in the diet. [11] Moreover, these protective effects are also seen in healthy populations. [11-15]

In healthy people with no evidence of heart disease, men and women appear to achieve the same level of protection against premature death by supplementing with omega 3 oils from fish and nuts. In a 2010 Norwegian study, elderly men with no evidence of heart disease who supplemented with fish oil experienced a 47% reduction in the risk of premature death, compared to those who did not supplement. [16]

Similarly, a large Australian study found that women with the highest levels of omega 3 consumption from nuts and fish had a 44% reduction in the risk of premature death from inflammatory disease. The protective effect was dose related to the level of omega 3 intake. [12] The ability of omega 3 fats to reduce the level of systemic inflammation through the production of anti-inflammatory prostaglandins (primitive cell-signalling hormones) appears to be the source of their protective talents.

There is abundant evidence that vitamin D prevents the proliferation of human breast cancer cells and enhances the differentiation of young cells into normal healthy tissue. [17-22] The risk of metastasis (spread) of breast cancer among women who have a deficiency in vitamin D at the time of diagnosis is almost double that of women with sufficient vitamin D stores. Vitamin D-deficient women also have a much greater risk of dying from this disease. Moreover, the risk of prostate cancer in men with low vitamin D status is triple that for men with sufficient vitamin D. [23-26] High blood levels of vitamin D have been shown to increase survival rates for colon cancer in both women and men by almost 50%. [27]

Iodine and iodine-rich foods have a long history of use in European and Asian cultures as natural remedies for cardiovascular disease and control of hypertension. [28-34] Textbooks from the mid 1900s advocate the use of iodides for the treatment of cardiovascular disorders, including arteriosclerosis, angina pectoris, aortic aneurism, and arterial hypertension. [35-37] The occurrence of iodine deficiency in cardiovascular disease is frequent. In people with thyroid disease, all cardiovascular abnormalities appear to be reversed by restoration of the normal thyroid state.[38] The documented antimicrobial, anti-inflammatory, and antiproliferative activities of iodine appear to be important factors in determining overall cardiovascular health.[39-42]

These studies and their findings are but a few of the thousands of independent scientific studies supporting the value of supplementation with higher quality nutritional supplements as a prudent, preventive measure for optimal health and disease prevention. Further evidence of the health-protective effects of nutritional supplementation will be discussed when we review two important and ancient antioxidants in the next chapter.

Media Spin

A New York Times article reporting on a 2006 Women's Health Initiative study disparaged the reported 29% reduction in fractures for those women who mostly stuck to their prescribed regimen as being only a "hint" of benefit.

It argued that to protect against osteoporosis women should consider, instead, taking several prescription drugs shown to prevent fractures.

The article, however, failed to mention that for some of these drugs the benefits are more modest than those obtained through simple vitamin D and calcium supplementation; for others, the drugs only work effectively when adequate vitamin D and calcium are present.

The Other Side
of the Coin

Certainly, the premise of life extension and disease prevention through supplementation does not have universal support amongst the scientific community. As is inevitably the case, in an evidence-based discipline there will arise conflicting studies that cast doubt on the evidence. Many researchers argue that supplements provide a convenient and effective means for supplying the optimal intakes of essential nutrients required to support long-term health; others counter that there is no conclusive proof that supplements provide any real health benefits at all.

Unfortunately, much of the debate is framed by a media more interested in selling newspapers than in ferreting out the truth. Sloppy reporting, distorted editorial sensationalism, and conflicts of interest by researchers and publishers have unnecessarily alarmed the public and have threatened to destroy public trust in complementary health care. Health-conscious consumers and medical practitioners alike have become frustrated at the mixed messages promulgated through the headlines: one day we are told something is good for us and the next day we are told it is not. Why do so many recently published studies appear to refute the prevailing scientific evidence about the benefits of natural approaches to wellness? How can vitamin E be good for us one day and bad for us the next? For once, why can't the experts just get it straight?

If there is any consolation, it may be helpful to understand that science never progresses smoothly; there will always be new findings that appear to refute long-established theories. Controversy is the crucible for change and the road that science must travel to arrive at a final truth. Unfortunately, media bias and conflicts of interest place unnecessary detours along the way.

Firstly, the consumer must understand that out of 100 clinical studies that investigate a particular effect probability dictates that five of these studies— no matter how well designed—will show results that are *not* real. There will always be a statistical fluke in the bunch.

Secondly, about one fifth of clinical trials investigating a particular effect will not have the needed number of subjects to show a statistically significant result. This occurs because in most clinical trials the probability of finding a real result, known as the power of a test, is set at a minimum of 80%. Consequently, there is up to a 20% chance of missing your mark and failing to find a difference when one actually exists. This is merely the gremlin of probability at work.

Thirdly, some investigations are just bad science, improperly conducted, poorly reported, and inadequately reviewed.

> The majority of clinical studies on the health benefits of natural health products continue to test individual supplements as though they are prescription drugs. This is not how vitamins work.

Unfortunately, as has been the case in numerous studies, their findings attract an inordinate amount of attention from a media hungry for headlines.

Poor Science, Poor Journalism—or Both?

A good example of one of these studies, which set the medical and scientific communities astir, is the 2005 Johns Hopkins University announcement that high-dose vitamin E can increase the risk of death among elderly patients.[43]

Here was a finding at complete odds with a surfeit of studies supporting the vitamin's long-established protective benefits.

The study was a meta-analysis, a statistically based methodology that combines the data from several published clinical trials. Properly done, a meta-analysis is a powerful investigative tool; mishandled, the results can be powerfully misleading. In selecting their studies for inclusion in the analysis, the authors disqualified several smaller investigations and those where there were fewer than 10 deaths reported in the trial. This served to introduce a sampling bias, which skewed the data to *support* the argument of harm. Moreover, many of the studies included in the analysis involved elderly subjects—many of whom were already seriously ill—rather than healthy adults. In one such trial, 31% (60)

of the subjects *died* during the study period. Nutritional intervention with gravely ill individuals can be a legitimate objective for a clinical study within a therapeutic context; however, applying the findings to the general population within the context of prevention is *not* legitimate.

On a final point, the studies included in the Johns Hopkins research used the synthetic *(d/l)* form of vitamin E. While there is no evidence of adverse effects from the consumption of the natural *(d)* form of vitamin E, the US National Academies of Science has long warned of adverse effects from taking high doses of synthetic vitamin E, including hemorrhagic toxicity, a serious and potentially fatal complication with elderly subjects who are already likely to be on blood thinners.

While publicly suggesting that high level intake of vitamin E may be dangerous, the authors, in their report, commented, "Overall, vitamin E supplementation did not affect all-cause mortality." The authors also duly reported that, at the highest dosages, the risk of death was actually *lower*—a finding that the media completely missed or chose to ignore.

So, what does the Johns Hopkins study actually reveal? First, the findings fail to make the case that high-dose vitamin E intake will increase the risk of death. More importantly, the study involved elderly people, many of whom were

gravely ill; therefore, whatever the findings, they simply *cannot* extend to the general, healthy population.

Unfortunately, when announcing their findings to the Press, the authors disregarded their own written guidance not to generalize the results, thus raising the spectre of harm to the public. The fallout was predictable: giving no consideration to the wealth of scientific evidence to the contrary, the Media took the bit at a full run, declaring that high-dose vitamin E may be deadly. Reacting with fear, consumers dumped vitamin E down the toilet by the truckload.

> **As instruments of wellness, natural health products generally lie outside the standard acute care model. For this reason, it is folly to evaluate the efficacy of such products and therapies through the looking glass of treatment/cure.**

To review more examples of these questionable studies, please refer to an investigative article written by this author for *Life Extension Magazine* (June, 2006) entitled *Media Bias, Conflicts of Interest Distort Study Findings on Supplements*. This review article is available at the following URL: *http://www.lef.org/magazine/mag2006/jun2006_cover_media_01.htm.*

Through the Looking Glass

Much of the controversy regarding the efficacy of nutritional supplements stems from peering through the lens of the prevailing drug-based model of treatment/

cure, the looking glass through which we evaluate the effectiveness of medical therapies. While this approach is certainly appropriate for drug products, it is entirely inappropriate for natural health products. Such products are, by nature, *preventive* rather than *curative*.

Within the drug-based model, the objective of most clinical trials is to evaluate a single drug for its therapeutic effect on a particular symptom or disease. Once a positive therapeutic effect is established, the drug is licensed for a specified treatment protocol. This *Magic Bullet* approach of high-tech, disease-centered medicine promises powerful, fast acting drugs that quickly produce therapeutic results. Unfortunately, it has absolutely *nothing* to do with prevention.

The drug-based approach is a disease-centered approach and the clinical trials employed by its adherents focus on treating already ill subjects. We call this secondary prevention—averting further progression of a disease that people already have. It is fundamentally different from that of primary prevention—thwarting the development of chronic disorders in a healthy population. Primary prevention is a lifelong undertaking to avoid disease, not a quick fix to rectify collateral damage from a poor lifestyle. Such an approach requires a *different* investigative lens.

> Vitamin E passes muster as an effective long-term measure for the *prevention* of heart disease, yet it fails the test when standard clinical trials evaluate its effectiveness as a *treatment* in patients with established disease.

Tragically, the majority of clinical studies on the health benefits of natural health products continue to test individual supplements as though they are prescription drugs, able to work in isolation and expected to provide dramatic health benefits over the short term in acutely ill people. This is *not* how vitamins work and, viewed within the paradigm of treatment/cure, it is no wonder they come up short.

For example, epidemiological and observational research supports the position that vitamin E, administered over the long term, helps prevent atherosclerosis (primary prevention). However, in a clinical setting vitamin E is ineffective in preventing the onset of a heart attack or stroke brought on by the rupture of an *existing* atherosclerotic plaque (secondary prevention). The findings of several clinical studies support this view. As such, vitamin E passes muster as an effective long-term measure for the *prevention* of heart disease, yet it fails the test when standard clinical trials evaluate its effectiveness as a *treatment* in patients with established disease.[44]

Does this mean that vitamin E is useless? Not at all. It simply demonstrates that the value of vitamin E as an agent in *prevention* is fundamentally different from its value as an agent of *intervention*.

As instruments of wellness, natural health products generally lie outside the standard acute care model. For this reason, it is folly to evaluate the efficacy of such products and therapies through the looking glass of treatment/cure. When evaluated within that paradigm they most often fail. These failures are subsequently paraded by the media as evidence that natural health products have no health benefits—cheered on by an international pharmaceutical cartel whose over-riding interest is to protect its bottom line.

Clearly, it is time for a new paradigm.

**Nothing makes sense in biology
except in the light of evolution.**

~ Theodosius Dobzhanski (1900 – 1975)
Evolutionary biologist and Orthodox Christian scholar

CHAPTER FIVE:

THE ANCIENT ANTIOXIDANTS

The exciting thing about the study of cellular biology is the perspective one gains from looking into the distant past. Only when peering through the lens of evolution do you gain a more complete understanding of the similarities between different life forms; only when parsing the biochemical mechanisms that empower all living systems do you more fully comprehend how *all* life shares a common origin.

Even the most advanced of organisms, the human species, had a simple beginning; the myriad biochemical processes that power human cells share a common ancestry with the simplest of creatures. This similarity can be observed when we investigate two nutrients that shared a common evolutionary path.

Vitamin D and iodine are ancient; their early biological roles as membrane antioxidants evolved concurrently as cellular life advanced. Today, these two life-giving nutrients act in a multitude of ways that are indispensable in maintaining cellular health.

In this chapter, we will explore a brief history of these ancient antioxidants to better understand how they came to play such fundamental roles in our health. We will also investigate some of the current research describing the protective effects of each. Lastly, we will highlight the fact that dietary deficiencies of both nutrients are the most pervasive and misunderstood global health challenges facing us today.

Vitamin D

~ a Brief History

So central is the role of vitamin D to the maintenance of life, we can trace its origins back to the unicellular zooplankton and phytoplankton that flourished in the ancient oceans over 750 million years ago—a time well before vertebrate life had evolved.[1] The vitamin's early evolutionary role as an antioxidant and its natural capacity to regulate calcium balance allowed early life forms to manufacture the necessary calcified skeletal structures that would later carry their successors onto land. *Emiliania huxleyi*, a photosynthetic phytoplankton with a global distribution from the tropics to the subarctic, is uniquely adorned with ornate calcite disks, a good example of an early life form that retains its capacity to manufacture vitamin D.

But vitamin D is not just about strong bones. While its core biochemical functions are inviolate, advancing life found other ways to harness vitamin D's talents, incorporating the nutrient into a growing number of cellular processes. Today, vitamin D plays a pivotal role in calcium balance, cell metabolism, gene expression, cell proliferation, cardiac health, immune function, and neurological support, and in tempering systemic inflammation.

Unlike other vitamins, vitamin D is not naturally found in substantial amounts in our food, other than fatty fish. A steroid hormone, it is manufactured in the outer layers of the skin through exposure to solar radiation. In this respect, it is not *truly* a vitamin (a vital food substance obtained from our diet) except in those individuals lacking sufficient sun exposure—which, in fact, is most of us.

Just as with the iguana, humans are built to obtain vitamin D through constant exposure to strong sunlight. That is why vitamin D is also known as the "sunshine vitamin."[2] The skin's ability to manufacture vitamin D is remarkable. Fifteen to thirty minutes of exposure to unprotected skin when the sun is high in the sky—enough to cause a slight 'pinkening' within 24 hours—is equivalent to taking 15,000-20,000 International Units (IU)[*] of vitamin D in supplement form.

Unfortunately, modern indoor lifestyles, the overuse of sunscreens (which filter out almost all the ultraviolet (UV) rays necessary to manufacture vitamin D), and seasonal variations in sun exposure do not provide us with sufficient natural stores of this important nutrient, particularly during the late fall and winter months. Because we *do not* obtain sufficient vitamin D from our diet alone, anyone living in a temperate climate *must* supplement with the sunshine vitamin or they will become deficient.

More than Just Strong Bones

Over the past several years, a flood of new research has revealed the extent of vitamin D's powers. Researchers have now discovered vitamin D receptors in *all* our body tissues. The hormone interacts with these receptors to elicit a multitude of physiological effects. That is why, when you think about it, your health and well-being depend heavily upon developing an intimate relationship with the sun.

Every tissue in the body has the enzymatic machinery to produce *activated* vitamin D (calcitriol)—*on the spot*—from the vitamin D reserves within. Once

---

[*] *The international unit is a unit of measurement for the amount of a substance based on the biological activity or effect. International units are used to quantify vitamins, hormones, some medications, vaccines, blood products, and similar biologically active substances.*

activated, calcitriol 'rolls up its sleeves,' interacting with receptors in the cell to regulate its growth and proliferation. Vitamin D's actions target over *2,000* genes in our cells, providing the hormone with an unprecedented degree of control over cellular function.

Working concurrently throughout the body and at the cellular level, vitamin D can: improve fertility; safeguard pregnancy; reduce chronic inflammation; help control weight; protect against infectious agents; help prevent strokes and neurological disorders, including dementia; bolster our immune response; boost mental cognition; modulate heart function; and support muscle strength[3]—all in all, not a bad day's work!

What we know, today, about vitamin D underscores the prophetic statement made decades ago by Nobel Laureate Dr Albert Szent-Györgyi: *Vitamins, if properly understood and applied, will help us to reduce suffering to an extent which the most fantastic human mind would fail to imagine.*

For most practitioners in mainstream medicine, it is simply incomprehensible that an ordinary vitamin can reduce the risks of heart attacks by as much as 50%; decrease the risks of cancers of the breast, colon, and prostate by a similar amount; reduce infectious diseases, including influenza, by as much as 90%; combat both type 1 and type 2 diabetes; diminish the risk of dementia and associated neurological dysfunctions; and impede the incidence of multiple sclerosis and other autoimmune diseases.[4]

But, this is no ordinary vitamin.

Vitamin D and Cancer

More than 2500 published studies confirm vitamin D's role in cancer prevention. Three of the most prevalent

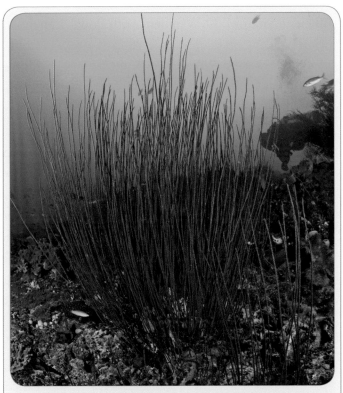

Figure 6: Vitamin D and Early Life Forms

Sea Whip (*Leptogorgia virgulata*) is a soft-bodied colonial coral with an internal skeleton found in the western Atlantic Ocean. This ancient organism is known to manufacture vitamin D as well as the iodine-containing hormone thyroxine.

and feared cancers—breast, colorectal, and prostate cancer—are highly influenced by the amount of sun exposure and vitamin D status. Research supports the position that supplementation with 1,000 IU per day or more of vitamin D will substantially reduce your risk of developing these cancers.

There is abundant evidence that vitamin D prevents the proliferation of human breast cancer cells and enhances the differentiation of young cells into normal healthy tissue.[5-10] The risk of metastasis (spread) of breast cancer among women who have a deficiency in vitamin D at the time of diagnosis is almost double that of women with sufficient vitamin D. Women with low vitamin D levels also have a much greater risk of dying from this disease. Moreover, the risk of prostate cancer in men deficient in vitamin D is triple that for men with sufficient vitamin D.[11-14] High blood levels of vitamin D have been shown to increase survival rates for colon cancer in both women and men by almost 50%.[15]

Twenty-five years of research suggests that high vitamin D intake may be especially important in averting colon cancer. A 19-year study of colorectal cancer rates found the relative risk in men with poor vitamin D status was almost triple that of men with sufficient vitamin D.[16] In a meta-analysis conducted on research worldwide from 1966 to 2004, researchers from the University of California concluded that 1,000 IU/day of vitamin D lowers an individual's risk of developing colorectal cancer by as much as 50%.[17]

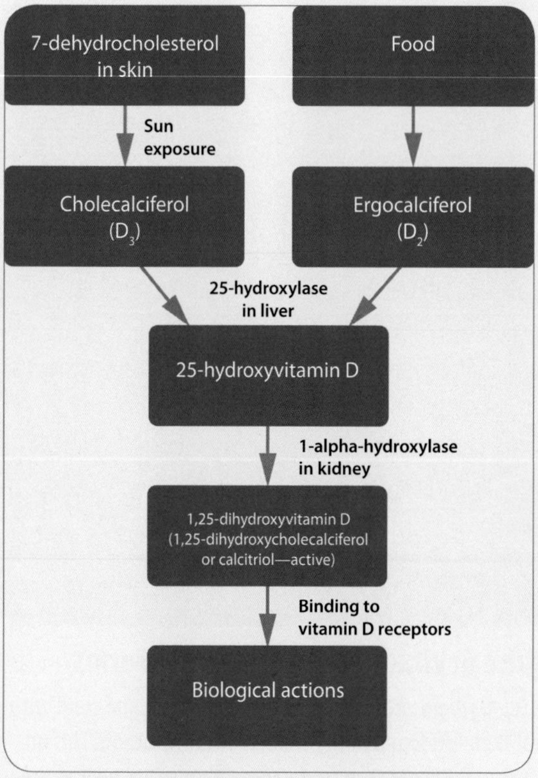

Epidemiological, ecological, and observational studies concur that the further away you live from the equator, the *poorer* is your vitamin D status and the *higher* is your lifetime risk of contracting cancer. While such studies, by design, cannot establish causality, findings dating back to 1941 confirm that cancer rates, including cancers of the breast, prostate, colon, ovaries, kidney, brain, pancreas, lung, and childhood cancers, are strongly correlated to latitude, solar intensity, and the lack of vitamin D.[11;12;18-29]

Circulating levels of vitamin D also play an important role in determining the outcomes of several cancers.

Figure 7: Vitamin D Synthesis

7-dehydrocholesterol in skin → (Sun exposure) → Cholecalciferol (D$_3$)

Food → Ergocalciferol (D$_2$)

→ (25-hydroxylase in liver) → 25-hydroxyvitamin D → (1-alpha-hydroxylase in kidney) → 1,25-dihydroxyvitamin D (1,25-dihydroxycholecalciferol or calcitriol—active) → (Binding to vitamin D receptors) → Biological actions

According to a 2009 review, support for the sunlight/vitamin D/cancer link is scientifically strong enough to warrant the use of vitamin D in cancer prevention and treatment protocols.[20] This view is widely supported by other scientists, some of who have called for mandatory vitamin D supplementation programs in countries where widespread insufficiency exists.[30]

In 2007, a four-year, population-based, double-blind, randomized, placebo-controlled trial—the gold standard for clinical trials—reported an astonishing finding. Postmenopausal women who supplemented with 1,100 IU/day of vitamin D and 1,500 mg/day of calcium reduced their risk of dying from ALL cancers by more than 66%, as compared to supplementing with calcium alone.[31] This remarkable finding has led some researchers to posit that vitamin D could be the *single* most effective means of preventing cancer—even outpacing the benefits of a healthy lifestyle.

According to Boston University's Dr Michael Holick, a recognized world authority on vitamin D, when you are exposed to strong sunlight or supplement with high levels of vitamin D, excess vitamin D is stored in your cellular tissues. This stored vitamin D can then be activated at any time to regulate abnormal cell growth that can lead to cancer. Once activated, vitamin D intervenes to halt the chaotic reproduction of precancerous cells by inducing *apoptosis*, a form of cellular

suicide. At the same time, the hormone inhibits the formation of new blood vessels needed to nourish cancerous growth—effectively snuffing out cancer *before* it takes hold.

This new understanding on how vitamin D can interfere with cancerous growth is the *singular* reason why scientists at the University of California, San Diego, now contend that low vitamin D status may be *the root cause* of all cancers.

Vitamin D and Heart Disease

The further north or south you live from the tropics, the higher is your risk of sudden death from a heart attack (myocardial infarction). A 1990 New Zealand study provided the first hint that vitamin D deficiency might be related to heart disease when researchers discovered seasonal variations in heart attacks that inversely mirrored similar cyclical variations in vitamin D status.[32] This finding was corroborated in a later US study that showed myocardial infarctions (MIs) surged by 53% during the winter months when sunlight and vitamin D production were low.[33] Conversely, in tropical climates the sun shines year-round and seasonal variations in the incidence of MI are not seen.[34]

In temperate climates lower light intensity during the winter months reduces vitamin D synthesis and encourages excess

> Vitamin D's benefits in stimulating general cardiovascular health are now recognized as being on par with that of aerobic exercise.

cholesterol synthesis, concurrently elevating the risks of atherosclerosis (plaque formation) and sudden heart attack.[35] A 2008 Harvard University study confirms that low vitamin D status can significantly increase the risk of a cardiac event in a *graded* manner.[36] Simply put, the *less* vitamin D you have in your blood, the *greater* is your risk of suddenly dropping dead.

People who are deficient in vitamin D are also much more likely to have high blood pressure (hypertension), type 2 diabetes, and elevated triglycerides (a major risk factor for heart disease) than people with normal levels of the sunshine vitamin.[37-39] Vitamin D reduces blood pressure by relaxing the smooth muscles lining artery walls and by regulating the release of renin, a hormone manufactured by the kidneys that increases vasoconstriction (constriction of the arteries).

As we learned in Chapter Two, C-reactive protein (CRP) is a principal biological marker of inflammation and heart disease, and a sensitive indicator of the risk of an impending cardiac event. As a potent anti-inflammatory agent, vitamin D has been found to effectively reduce levels of CRP.[40] The ability of vitamin D to reduce CRP appears to be even more pronounced than that of the statin drugs commonly used by the pharmaceutical industry to reduce the risk of heart attack.[41] Additionally, the vitamin's benefits in stimulating general cardiovascular health are now recognized

as being on par with that of aerobic exercise. A deficiency of vitamin D diminishes the contractile function of the heart, contributes to dysfunction in the endothelial lining of the blood vessels, worsens fatty plaque formation, and contributes to congestive heart failure.[42-44]

Vitamin D status is also inversely related to the risk of deep vein thrombosis, a dangerous clotting of the major veins in the legs that can lead to acute pulmonary embolism* and sudden death. The findings of a 2009 Swedish study on thrombosis are similar to the New Zealand and US studies on heart attacks and indicate that the risks of thrombotic complications display a seasonal variation, peaking in the winter months and dropping in the summer. High levels of vitamin D appear to enhance the blood's anticlotting capacity and reduce both inflammation and the risk of clot formation.[45]

Researchers now understand that inflammation of the arteries is a major contributory factor in congestive heart failure. Vitamin D offers protective benefits to the endothelial cells lining the arteries and heart muscle by quelling the production of inflammatory proteins that contribute to heart failure. The authors of a recent German study conclude that supplemental vitamin D could serve as a new anti-inflammatory agent for the treatment of this disease.[46]

---

* *A pulmonary embolism is a sudden blockage in the pulmonary artery of the lung (or one of its branches) resulting from dislodged clotted fragments (embolisms) that migrate in the blood through the body.*

Vitamin D and Immune Support

For years, the evidence has mounted that sun exposure is an effective prevention and treatment for immune disorders. Like cancer and heart disease, the prevalence of these disorders correlates directly with latitude and is demonstrated dutifully each year when the waning sunlight of autumn presages the onslaught of the flu season.

Researchers now believe that seasonal colds and influenza may actually be the result of *decreased* levels of vitamin D, rather than of *increased* wintertime viral activity.[47] Several studies reveal that vitamin D is required for proper activation of specialized immune cells responsible for killing harmful viruses and bacteria.[48;49] The strength of the evidence supporting vitamin D's efficacy in reducing viral-borne infections has convinced many physicians to recommend boosting daily intakes of vitamin D

to 5,000 IU per day or more during the flu season, rather than submit to the risks and questionable effectiveness of flu shots.

A previously unexpected role for vitamin D in bolstering our natural immunity has been documented by researchers at the University of California, San Diego: keratinocytes, the predominant cells in the outer layer of skin, can independently activate vitamin D from within their stores. Once activated, vitamin D switches on selected genes controlling the manufacture of *cathelicidin*, a specialized antimicrobial protein that specifically targets viruses, bacteria, and other infectious agents.[50] This enables skin cells to *directly* respond to the presence of microbes and protect wounds against infection.

Vitamin D also demonstrates protective benefits in autoimmune dysfunctions. Diseases such as lupus, fibromyalgia, type 1 diabetes (an autoimmune disease of the pancreas), psoriasis, rheumatoid arthritis, chronic fatigue syndrome, and multiple

Table 2: Recommendations for Daily Intake of Vitamin D
From: Holick MF, *The Vitamin D Solution*, Hudson Street Press, 2010, p 219

AGE OR CONDITION	INTAKE PER DAY	SAFE UPPER LIMIT
Infants 0 to 1 yr	400-1,000 IU	2,000 IU
Children 1 yr to 12 yrs	1,000-2,000 IU	5,000 IU
Adolescents 13+ and adults	1,500-2,000 IU	10,000 IU
Obese individuals of any age	2-3 times the above	10,000 IU
Pregnant women	1,400-2,000 IU	10,000 IU
Lactating women*	2,000-4,000 IU	10,000 IU

* Lactating women who want to ensure their baby is getting sufficient vitamin D from their breast milk should supplement with 4,000 – 6,000 IU/day

sclerosis are some of the common auto-immune diseases related to impaired vitamin D status.[51] Recent studies reveal that vitamin D may temper the overstimulation of our immune system and help reduce *both* allergic and autoimmune responses. One of the mechanisms appears to be vitamin D's ability to directly inhibit the activation of nuclear factor-kappa beta (Nf-kB), the master switch that controls the body's inflammatory cascade.[52-54] (To review information on Nf-kB, please turn to Chapter Two.)

Indeed, vitamin D's immune-bolstering talents make it one of our most reliable nutritional tools in augmenting comprehensive immunity. Scientists and medical experts throughout Europe, Canada, the United States, and elsewhere have called for a global policy change on vitamin D, which they contend is crucial to reduce the risks of a host of degenerative diseases.

The Bottom Line

Despite the rapid advancement in our knowledge about vitamin D, chronic insufficiency of this vital nutrient remains one of today's most unrecognized and misdiagnosed global health challenges. More than one billion people worldwide remain chronically deficient in vitamin D. Tragically, calls to increase the recommended daily intake of vitamin D to 1,000 IU/day or more for adults have gone largely unheeded. Marginal improvements in the recommended daily intakes of 600 IU/day, issued in 2010 by the United States and Canada, appear insufficient to address the problem. Vitamin D authority Dr Michael Holick proposes that a daily dose of between 1,000–2,000 IU/day is a necessary preventive measure for everyone. Holick further contends that doses between 2,000 to 5,000 IU/day are perfectly safe over the long term.[55]

Iodine ~ a Brief History

Much like its nutritional colleague vitamin D, iodine is another of our most fundamental yet misunderstood nutrients. A simple element of the halogen chemical family, iodine is found principally in the form of highly soluble iodide (I^{-1}_{aq}), which concentrates in oceans, brine pools, and subterranean water sources. Free iodine occurs mainly in its volatile molecular form as I_2, after being oxidized from iodide. A relatively rare element on land, its ubiquity in the world's oceans, its fat solubility, and its ability to participate in oxidative reactions made iodine the perfect candidate for a cellular antioxidant during early evolution.

Cyanobacteria,* which arose early in the ancient seas, developed a strong affinity for iodine. These primitive bacteria appear to have incorporated iodine's talents as

---

* *An ancient form of photosynthetic bacteria (blue-green algae) found in almost every terrestrial and aquatic habitat, cyanobacteria are responsible for the earth's early production of free molecular oxygen.*

an antioxidant to quench toxic oxygen free radicals generated during photosynthesis.[56] Kelp, another early marine life form, is known to actively scavenge iodine from the surrounding waters when placed under oxidative stress, presumably for the same reason.

Over millions of years, iodine's initial role as a membrane antioxidant and its ability to spontaneously couple with the amino acid tyrosine allowed the creation of a highly reactive and mobile species, *iodotyrosine*. Iodinated tyrosine was later incorporated into evolving biochemical pathways for energy production, gene expression, and DNA replication. Further conversions of iodotyrosine gave rise to thyroxine (T4) and triiodothyronine (T3), powerful hormones that, today, are manufactured in the thyroid glands of advanced vertebrates.[57] The thyroid gland exerts considerable control over the body, determining how it uses energy, manufactures proteins, and regulates sensitivity to the actions of other hormones. Not surprisingly, invertebrates and algae continue to possess the ability to synthesize thyroxine, presumably to fulfill similar needs.[58]

Within the thyroid gland, and apart from its role in the manufacture of hormones, iodine's antioxidant clout protects thyroid cells from the oxidative burden that is the very *nature* of thyroid hormone synthesis. The manufacture of hydrogen peroxide is the hallmark of thyroid physiology and its production during hormone synthesis places the thyroid under a heavy oxidative load.[59] With sufficient iodide present, the reactive-oxygen free radicals produced are effectively removed and cellular damage is averted. Until recently, medical science believed that the only tissue requiring iodine was the thyroid gland—we now know, this is not the case.

More than Just the Thyroid

Up to 70% of the body's iodine is stored in several other tissues, including breast, thymus gland, eyes, gastric mucosa, cervix, arteries, bones, joints, and salivary glands. Iodine's presence at these sites is so critical, the cells of these tissues have developed a specific mechanism, known as the sodium iodide symporter (a type of molecular pump), to actively transport the element across a membrane concentration gradient as high as 50-fold.[60]

Iodine is a powerful biological antioxidant. Painted on the skin, tincture of iodine will destroy 90% of the surface bacteria within 90 seconds. Paradoxically, while toxic to other bacteria, the development of iodine's *protective* antioxidant role in cyanobacteria helped make photosynthesis and the later evolution of oxygen-breathing life forms possible.

In breast and other tissues, elemental iodide (I$^-$) donates electrons to hydrogen peroxide to form iodinated proteins and lipids and to reduce damaging free radical formation.[61] Within the blood, iodide actively scours other free radicals. Within the salivary glands and breast tissues, it attaches to unsaturated fats in the cell membranes to protect them from autocatalytic (self-perpetuating) peroxidation. The high iodide concentration of the thymus gland supports the important antioxidant role of iodine in the immune system.[61]

This simple element, abundant in the ancient seas and incorporated as an antioxidant in the earliest of living cells, now plays an indispensable role in human physiology and health.

Iodine Deficiency

While the primary manifestation of iodine deficiency is goitre, a nodular swelling of the thyroid gland, it is only the most visible sign. There are several other consequences, including hearing loss, learning deficits, brain damage, and myelination disorders, that can occur during foetal development.[62] One of the most devastating of these iodine deficiency disorders is congenital hypothyroidism, which often leads to cretinism and irreversible mental retardation.[63] In women, iodine deficiency can lead to overt hyperthyroidism, anovulation, infertility, gestational hypertension, spontaneous abortion, and stillbirths.[64]

Mild hypothyroidism* in pregnant women has been associated with marked cognitive impairment in their offspring.[65;66] There is also a greater prevalence of attention deficit disorders (ADD) amongst the offspring of mothers from iodine-deficient regions compared to those in marginally deficient regions. In a 2004 study, researchers showed that 69% of the offspring from iodine-deficient areas were diagnosed as attention deficit hyperactivity disorder (ADHD)—an austere contrast to the 0% diagnosed in marginally deficient areas.[67]

Researchers focusing on iodine's role in cardiovascular health have found that changes in thyroid status influence cardiac contractile and electrical activity.[68] The iodine-containing hormones manufactured by the thyroid are important metabolic regulators of cardiovascular activity; they have the ability to exert action on the myocardium (heart muscles), the vascular smooth muscles, and the endothelium.† As well, recent evidence supports iodine's role in controlling insulin and blood-sugar levels in diabetics.[69-71]

Iodine and Cancer

Today, one in seven women in North America will develop breast cancer in their lifetime. Thirty years ago—when iodine consumption was double what it is now‡—only one in 20 women developed the disease.[56] In reviewing epidemiological studies of breast cancer, researchers have

---

* Hypothyroidism is a common endocrine disorder that occurs when the thyroid produces insufficient levels of T3 and T4 hormones. Insufficient dietary iodine is the most common cause of hypothyroidism.

† The endothelium is the thin layer of cells that lines the interior surfaces of blood and lymphatic vessels. It forms a protective interface between circulating blood or lymph and the rest of the vessel wall.

concluded that there appears to be a *single* reputed factor protective against breast cancer—one that is lipid soluble—the depletion of which is responsible for the vast majority of cases.[72] It is generally believed that this protective factor is the element iodine.[73-77] The ductal cells of the breast, the ones most likely to turn cancerous, are known to contain the sodium iodide symporter, allowing these cells to sequester iodine from the blood and maintain high levels of the nutrient within cellular tissues.

Studies on iodine and breast cancer highlight a close correlation with insufficient iodine levels and malignant growth. Canadian scientists have proposed a facilitating role for iodine in reducing the cancer-promoting effects of oestrogen and in maintaining the normalization of breast tissues.[75;78] Breast cancer patients express decidedly lower levels of iodine in their breast tissues than do healthy subjects.[79] Chronic iodine insufficiency has been found to alter both the structure and function of the mammary glands, especially the alveolar cells, which sequester

iodine at high levels. Iodine at 5 mg daily has been found to reduce the size of both benign and malignant breast tumours, an effect credited to the nutrient's capacity to reduce autocatalytic lipid peroxidation.

Importantly, iodine has also been shown to induce apoptosis in abnormal breast tissue. This process of programmed cell death is essential for proper growth and development. In the foetus, for example, apoptosis allows for the degradation of nonessential tissues, such as the webbing between the toes and fingers that occurs during gestation. In the same manner, apoptosis destroys precancerous cells that have come to represent a threat to the integrity of the organism.[80] This unique anticancer

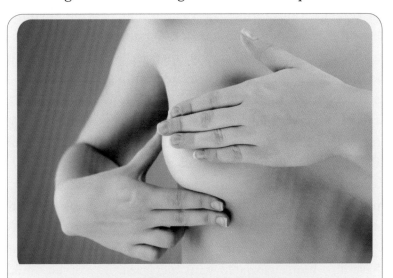

Figure 8: Breast Self-examination
Regular self-examination of breast architecture is an important preventive measure for reducing the risk of metastatic breast cancer.

‡ *The liberal use of iodized salt was encouraged during the early to mid 1900s as a means of reducing thyroid disease. This had the unfortunate and unintended consequence of increasing the levels of hypertension and cardiovascular disease. The consequent reduction in the consumption of iodized salt, our principal source of iodine in modern times, has resulted in a concurrent drop in iodine.*

function of iodine may well prove to be its most important extrathyroidal benefit.

Several studies highlight the ability of iodine to induce apoptosis in both animal and human cancer-cell lines.[81-83] Iodine's ability to induce cell death appears to be a function of its concentration in these tissues. In the first report demonstrating that a therapeutic dose of iodide is effective and highly selective against lung cancer, the authors demonstrated that increasing the intracellular levels of iodide in lung cancer cells killed greater than 95% of the aberrant cells.[81]

People living in iodine-deficient areas are not only prone to thyroid disorders, they also experience a higher incidence of stomach cancer. Like the thyroid and breast, the cells lining the stomach contain a rich concentration of iodine. Increased iodine intake is strongly correlated with a reduction in the incidence of stomach cancer.[84] In Poland, which has one of the highest incidences of stomach cancer in the world, researchers observed a strong association between improved iodine supply and a decrease in the incidence of stomach cancer.[84]

Deficiencies of this essential nutrient have also been associated with increased risk for thyroid, prostate, endometrial, and ovarian cancers.[85-90] Furthermore, there is a *strong* correlation between iodine insufficiency and the development of fibrocystic breast disease as well as breast cancer.[63] The strength of the evidence is so compelling that researchers hypothesize these

diseases may, like goitre and cretinism, be iodine-deficiency disorders.[80]

Iodine and Heart Health

Iodine and iodine-rich foods have a long history of use in European and Asian cultures as natural remedies for cardiovascular disease and control of hypertension.[91-97] Medical textbooks from the mid 1900s advocate the use of iodides for the treatment of cardiovascular disorders, including arteriosclerosis, angina pectoris, aortic aneurism, and arterial hypertension.[98-100]

The occurrence of iodine deficiency in cardiovascular disease is frequent. In people with thyroid disease, all cardiovascular abnormalities appear to be reversed by restoration of the normal thyroid state.[101] The documented antimicrobial, anti-inflammatory, and antiproliferative activities of iodine appear to be important factors in determining overall cardiovascular health.[68;102-104] Moreover, iodine's ability to reduce blood viscosity facilitates a measurable reduction in blood pressure and lowers the accompanying risk of an adverse cardiac event.[104]

Even mild hypothyroidism contributes to cardiovascular disease and stroke. Thyroid failure, which is generally a consequence of chronic iodine insufficiency, also contributes to the development of coronary artery disease.[105-107] In one study, individuals with subclinical hyperthyroidism exhibited a 41% increase in mortality from all causes, compared to normal subjects.[108] Thyroid dysfunction induced by iodine deficiency can elevate low-density lipoproteins (LDL cholesterol) and total cholesterol and can raise the risk of atherosclerosis. As well, the effect of insufficient iodine on cardiovascular function can be characterized by decreased myocardial contractility and increased peripheral vascular resistance. Iodine deficiency can also weaken the contractile function of the heart muscle and can create life threatening cardiac arrhythmias—an effect that may become dangerously pronounced during even moderate exercise.[106]

Relatively low thyroid function is also associated with more severe blockage of the coronary and carotid arteries and impaired endothelial function.[109-112] Supporting studies show that the iodine-containing hormones T3 and T4 influence the cardiovascular system through their direct actions on vascular smooth muscles, cardiac muscle, kidney function, haemostasis (blood clotting), and alteration of homocysteine* levels.[113-117] Consequently, restoring normal thyroid function through iodine supplementation can help reverse a *multitude* of cardiovascular risk factors.[105;118;119]

> Unless you eat copious amounts of seaweed and other marine plant species, or sprinkle unhealthy amounts of iodized salt on your meal, iodine is not easily obtainable from your food.

Iodine and Breast Health

Perhaps the most compelling evidence of an extrathyroidal role for iodine is its impact on breast health. Sufficient dietary iodine is critical in maintaining breast health, a relationship that has been documented for well over a century. Chronic iodine deficiency causes fibrocystic breast disease (FBD), with characteristic nodules, cyst formation, pain, and scarring. A 1928 US-based autopsy series reported a 3% incidence of FBD; by 1973, the incidence of this disease had exploded to 89% of the female population, plausibly in direct relation to steadily decreasing levels of iodine intake.[71] According to a 2001 report by the American Cancer Society, 90% of the women examined at that time displayed benign breast changes, including lumps and tumours, when examined microscopically.[120]

Next to the thyroid gland, the breasts are the main glandular storage organ for iodine. Breast tissue has a high affinity for iodine, which is required for normal growth and development of proper breast architecture.[121] When tissue stores are

---

* *Homocysteine is a sulfur-containing amino acid that can elevate oxidative damage in the cardiovascular system. High levels of homocysteine are known to elevate the risks of cardiovascular disease and cardiac events.*

replete, iodine acts as an antioxidant and antiproliferative agent, protecting the integrity of the breast tissue.[122] As an antioxidant, iodine targets hydrogen peroxide, peroxidase and unsaturated membrane lipids in the breast, thereby decreasing oxidative damage to breast tissue cells.[123]

Human breast tissue and breast milk are rich sources of iodine, much greater than the thyroid gland itself.[62;124] In fact, human breast milk contains a concentration of iodine four times greater than thyroid tissue, indicative of the high biological demand for iodine by the nursing infant. Breast tissue is also rich in the same globular iodine-transporting proteins used by the thyroid to sequester iodine from the blood, indicating a clear evolutionary need for iodine in neonatal care. As mentioned previously, the element is vital for the proper neurological development of the newborn; consequently, nature has developed a direct means of nourishing and protecting the infant with this essential nutrient.[125]

The Bottom Line

Iodine deficiency is considered to be the most common glandular disorder and the most preventable cause of mental retardation worldwide. Fully one third of the world's population—more than 2 billion people—live in iodine-deficient areas.[126;127] Nowadays, about 800 million people are affected by iodine deficiency diseases that include goitre, hypothyroidism, mental retardation, and other growth and developmental abnormalities.[128] Despite the fact that infant mortality rates have been shown to plummet wherever iodine deficiencies have been eliminated, maternal iodine deficiencies during pregnancy and postnatal development continue to place millions of the world's children at risk—a tragic situation that is easily and entirely preventable.[62]

Unless you eat copious amounts of seaweed and other marine plant species, or sprinkle unhealthy amounts of iodized salt on your meal, iodine is not easily obtainable from your food. For that reason, it is important to complement your diet with an iodine-containing nutritional supplement to ensure your daily intake requirements are met. Current recommended intakes of 150 micrograms per day (μg/day) are now seen as insufficient. Several researchers emphasize that a daily iodine intake of up to 1 mg (1,000 μg) or more is needed to support other cellular functions.

Facts are the air of scientists.
Without them you can never fly.

~ Linus Pauling (1901-1994)
Nobel Laureate in Chemistry and Peace

CHAPTER SIX:

COMPARING SUPPLEMENTS

Every nutritional product included in the *NutriSearch Comparative Guide to Nutritional Supplements™* is assigned a rating based on a comprehensive analytical model developed by NutriSearch. This model is based on a compilation of the recommended daily nutritional intakes of 12 independent nutritional authorities. Each of the 12 authorities cited has published one or more works that recommend specific daily nutritional intakes deemed important for long-term health. Each author, listed below, is acknowledged within his or her respective scientific, medical, and naturopathic field:

Robert Atkins, MD: The late Robert Atkins was the founder and medical director of the Atkins Center for Complementary Medicine in New York City. An early proponent of the value of nutritional supplementation, Dr Atkins' bestselling book, *Dr Atkins' Vita-Nutrient Solution,* stresses the importance of daily supplementation in overcoming nutritional deficiencies found in our foods today. A practising physician and a professor of medicine at Capital University

of Integrative Medicine, Dr Atkins gained recognition in 1972 with the publication of his first book, *Dr Atkins' Diet Revolution.* Subsequent to this, he wrote *Dr Atkins' Nutrition Breakthrough* and *Dr Atkins' Health Revolution.*

Phyllis Balch, CNC: Until her death in 2004, Phyllis Balch was a leading nutritional consultant, recognized for her expertise in nutrition-based therapies. She authored several bestselling books, including: *Prescription for Dietary Wellness: Using Foods to Heal; Prescription for Herbal Healing: An Easy-to-Use A-Z Reference to Hundreds of Common Disorders and Their Herbal Remedies;* and *Prescription for Nutritional Healing: the A-to-Z Guide to Supplements,* coauthored by **Dr James Balch**, a certified urologist, a member of the American Medical Association, and a Fellow of the American College of Surgeons. Because of the coauthorship of *Prescription for Nutritional Healing [2002],* on which we base their recommendations, we recognize the authors as a single reference source.

Michael Colgan, PhD, CCN: Dr Colgan is a bestselling author and internationally acclaimed speaker on antiaging, sports nutrition, and hormonal health. His first public book, *Your Personal Vitamin Profile,* was considered a definitive guide for accurate, scientifically researched nutritional information. He has subsequently authored *Hormonal Health: Nutritional and Hormonal Strategies for Emotional Well-Being and Intellectual Longevity* and *The New Nutrition: Medicine for the Millennium.* Dr Colgan has served as a consultant to the US National Institute on Aging and to the US, Canadian, and New Zealand governments as well as to many corporations. His professional memberships include the New York Academy of Sciences, the American Academy of Anti-Aging Medicine, the American College of Sports Medicine, and the British Society for Nutritional Medicine. In 2002, Dr Colgan was inducted into the Canadian Nutrition Hall of Fame. In 2011, Dr Colgan partnered with Isagenix International, joining with their scientific research team to find nutritional products that would help slow aging.

Terry Grossman, MD and Ray Kurzweil are coauthors of *Fantastic Voyage,* an insightful book on the science behind radical life extension. Dr Grossman is the founder and medical director of Frontier Medical Institute in Denver, Colorado. A diplomat of the American Board of Chelation Therapy (ABCT) and a member of the American Academy for Advancement of Medicine (ACAM), the International Oxidative Medicine Association (IOMA), and the American Academy of Anti-aging Medicine (A4M), Dr Grossman is a licensed homeopathic and a naturopathic medical doctor; he now runs the Grossman Health and Wellness Center in Denver, Colorado. **Ray Kurzweil** is one of the world's leading inventors, thinkers and futurists. He is the author of three previous books, *The Age of Spiritual Machines; The 10% Solution for a Healthy Life;* and *The Age of Intelligent Machines.* Kurzweil received the 1999 National Medal of Technology; in 2002, he was inducted into the National Inventor Hall of Fame. Named Honorary Chairman for Innovation of the White House Conference on Small Business by President Reagan in 1986, he has received additional honours from former Presidents Clinton and Johnson.

Jane Higdon, PhD: With over 13 years of experience as a certified family nurse practitioner, Jane Higdon also held a Master of Science in nursing, a Master of Science in exercise physiology, and a Doctorate in nutrition. Until her tragic death in 2006, Jane Higdon was a Research Associate at the Linus Pauling Institute, Oregon State University. The Linus Pauling Institute's mission is to determine the function and role of micronutrients and phytochemicals in promoting optimum health and in preventing and treating disease. The Institute conducts research to determine the role of oxidative stress and antioxidants in human health and disease.

Philip Lee Miller, MD and Life Extension Foundation are coauthors of *The Life Extension Revolution: The New Science of Growing Older Without Aging* (2005). Dr Miller is the founder and medical director of the California Age Management Institute, Los Gatos, California. A practising physician for over 30 years, he is a diplomat of the American Board of Anti-Aging Medicine and serves on the Medical Advisory Board of **Life Extension Foundation (LEF)**, the world's largest organization dedicated to the science of preventing and treating degenerative disease and aging. In addition to developing unique disease treatment protocols, LEF funds pioneering scientific research aimed at achieving an extended healthy lifespan. At the heart of Life Extension's mission are its research programs for identifying and developing new therapies to slow and reverse the deterioration associated with aging.

Earl Mindell, RPh, MH has written 48 books on nutrition and health, including the bestseller, *Dr Mindell's Vitamin Bible*, published in the mid 1980s. Subsequent publications include *Earl Mindell's Vitamin Bible for the 21st Century*; *Dr Mindell's What You Should Know About Creating Your Own Personal Health Plan*; *Earl Mindell's Herb Bible*;

Earl Mindell's Food as Medicine; *Shaping up with Vitamins*; and *Earl Mindell's Anti-Aging Bible*. Mindell received a Bachelor of Science in Pharmacy in 1964, earning his Master's in Herbal Medicine in 1995. He is a registered pharmacist and a Fellow of the British Institute of Homeopathy.

Michael Murray, ND is one of the world's leading authorities on natural medicine. He has published over 30 books featuring natural approaches to health. In addition to his private practice as a consultant to the health food industry, he has been instrumental in bringing many effective natural products to North America. His research into the health benefits of proper nutrition is the foundation for a bestselling line of dietary supplements from Natural Factors, where he is Director of Product Development. He is a graduate, former faculty member, and serves on the Board of Regents of Bastyr University in Seattle, Washington.

Richard Passwater, PhD has been a research biochemist since 1959. His first areas of research interest were in the development of pharmaceuticals, spectrophotoluminescence and analytical chemistry. He has continued to research nutritional supplements and has now published over 42 books and booklets, as well as over 500 articles on nutrition and nutritional supplements. Twice honoured by the Committee for World Health, his scientific contributions have garnered him worldwide recognition. His discovery of biological antioxidant synergism in 1962 has been the focus of his research since that time. In 1973, Dr Passwater's article *Cancer: New Directions* was the first to report that a synergistic combination of antioxidant nutrients significantly reduces cancer incidence. His pioneering work with Drs Linus Pauling and James Enstrom highlighted the protective effect of vitamin E against heart disease. His bestselling book, *Supernutrition: Megavitamin Revolution,*   legitimized   megavitamin therapy. Dr Passwater's most recent public books include *The Antioxidants; The New Supernutrition;* and *Cancer Prevention and Nutritional Therapies.* He is the nutrition editor for *The Experts Journal of Optimal Health* and the scientific editor for *Whole Foods,* and he serves on the editorial board of the *Journal of Applied Nutrition.* Dr Passwater is also the Director of the Solgar Nutritional Research Center.

Nicholas   Perricone,   MD is   a board-certified   clinical   and   research dermatologist.   An   internationally recognized   antiaging   expert,   award-winning inventor, and a respected scientific researcher, Dr Perricone is an Adjunct Professor of Medicine at the Michigan State University's College of Human Medicine. Certified by the American Board of Dermatology, he is also a Fellow of the New York Academy of Sciences, the American College of Nutrition, the American Academy of Dermatology, and the Society of Investigative Dermatology. Dr Perricone has served as Assistant Clinical Professor of Dermatology at Yale School of Medicine and as Chief of Dermatology at Connecticut's Veterans Hospital. He is author of *The Perricone Weight-loss Diet* and *The Acne Prescription* and has written three New York Times bestsellers: *The Wrinkle Cure; The Perricone Prescription;* and *The Perricone Promise.*

Ray Strand, MD has practised family medicine for four decades, focussing over the past 20 years on nutritional medicine. An articulate advocate for the integration of   optimal   nutrition   and   advanced nutritional   therapies   in   preventive healthcare, he is a member of the Scientific Advisory Board of Ariix, a premier health and   wellness   company.   Dr   Strand   has lectured   on   nutritional   medicine   across the United States, Canada, Australia, New Zealand, and England. His publications include *Bionutrition: Winning   the   War Within; Death by Prescription; Healthy for Life; What Your Doctor Doesn't Know About Nutritional Medicine May Be Killing You; Preventing Diabetes;* and *Living by Design.*

Julian   Whitaker,   MD is   the   author of   several   popular   books,   including *Reversing   Diabetes;   Reversing   Heart Disease;* and *Dr Whitaker's Guide to Natural Healing.* Board   certified   in   antiaging medicine, Dr Whitaker belongs to the American College for Advancement in Medicine   and   is   a   founding   member of the American Preventive Medicine Association. He became fascinated early in his career by the preventive and healing powers of nutrition and natural therapies. In 1974, along with four other heathcare professionals and two-time Nobel Prize winner Linus Pauling, Dr Whitaker founded the California Orthomolecular Medical Society. In 1976, he joined the staff at the Pritikin Longevity Center, and in 1979 he founded the Whitaker Wellness Institute. Today, Whitaker Wellness is the largest alternative medicine clinic in the United States, where patients participate in an intensive program of diet, exercise, nutritional and herbal supplementation, and lifestyle change.

In borrowing from the preceding authors' scientific insights to construct our analytical standard, we recognize the immense contribution that they have made, individually and collectively, to the advancement of scientific knowledge and the pursuit of optimal health.

The Blended Standard

The individual recommendations for daily nutrient intakes from the 12 authorities cited above are pooled to construct the *Blended Standard*, the measure by which every product in the *NutriSearch Comparative Guide to Nutritional Supplements™* is compared. While each author's recommendations may have characteristics not recognized by the others, we have exploited their substantial commonality. Unless otherwise noted, for a nutrient to qualify for inclusion in the *Blended Standard*, three of the 12

authorities must cite a recommended daily intake for the specified nutrient. In all, 47 nutrient categories, consisting of 19 vitamins or vitamin-like factors, 13 minerals, five phytonutrient complexes, three omega fatty acids, and seven other nutritional factors are identified and incorporated into the standard.

The recommended daily intake for each nutrient is determined, wherever possible, by calculating the median (middle) value from those authors who provide a specific dosage recommendation. In some cases, where recent scientific evidence has eclipsed the recommendations, *NutriSearch* provides a recommended daily intake— or removes a previously recommended nutrient—based upon these new findings. Since the 2007 (4ᵗʰ Edition) of the guide, modifications have been made to the pooled recommendations in two key areas based upon new scientific findings. This includes changes to the daily levels of intake of the following:

✔ Vitamin D has been increased from 400IU/day to 1,000 IU/day
✔ Iodine has been increased from 100 µg/day to 1,000 µg/day

With the exception of Passwater's recommendations (which are based on diet, level of health, and physical activity), the recommended daily intakes published by each author are presented for the general adult population. Passwater's lower two categories (C and D) are selected for

Continued on page 65

Table 3: Table of Recommended Daily Intakes (Blended Standard)

Nutritional Components	Amt	Atkins Average	Balch/Balch Average	Colgan Average	Higdon/LPI Average	Grossman/Kurzweil Average	Miller/LEF Average	Mindell Average	Murray Average	Passwater Average	Perricone Average	Strand Average	Whitaker Average	Blended Standard Median	NOTES	Upper Limits (UL)
Vitamins																
Vitamin A	IU	2,250	7,500	6,250	5,000	5,000	5,000	NR	5,000	17,500		NR	5,000	5,000		10,000 IU
Vitamin D	IU	135	400	400	600	1,300	400	300	250	650		625	250	1,000	†	2000 IU
Vitamin K	ug		300	75	no amt	105	7,500	180	180			75	180	180		ND
B-Complex Vitamins																
Biotin	ug	338	600	500	30	600	300	200	200	63		650	200	250		ND
Folic Acid	ug	3,000	600	400	400		800	350	400	600		900	300	600		1000 ug
Vitamin B1 (thiamin)	mg	45	75	50	2	105	100	38	55	63		25	55	55		ND
Vitamin B2 (riboflavin)	mg	36	33	45	2	55	50	63	30	63		38	55	45		ND
Vitamin B3 (niacin)	mg	23	33	50	20	60	50	63	55	63		53	55	[28]		35 mg
Vitamin B3 (niacinamide)	mg	45	75	80			150		20					60		ND
Vitamin B5 (pantethine)	mg	113												ID		ND
Vitamin B5 (pantothenic acid)	mg	113	75	150	10		400	63	63	150		140	63	75		ND
Vitamin B6 (pyridoxine)	mg	45	75	50	2	75	50	100	63	63		38	63	63		100 mg
Vitamin B6 (pyridoxyl-5-phosphate)	mg	9												ID		ND
Vitamin B12 (cobalamin)	ug	210	300	100	18	18	100	550	400	88		175	300	175		ND
Antioxidant Vitamins and Nutrients																
Coenzyme Q10	mg		65	30		130	125	60	100	35	30	25		60		ND
alpha-Lipoic acid	mg			100		150	375		35		28	23		100		ND
para-Aminobenzoic Acid	mg	450	30		300		50			63				NR		ND
Vitamin C	mg	750	2,000	2,000	200	1,250	3,000	2,000	1,000	7,000		1,500	175	1,500		2000 mg
Vitamin E (as alpha tocopherol)	IU	225	500	400	299	600	1,000	400	600	700		600	600	600		1467 IU (1000 mg)
Vitamin E (as gamma tocopherol or mixed tocopherols)	mg			200										200	^^^	ND
Bioflavonoid Complex																
Bioflavonoids (mixed/citrus)	mg	525	350	350					4,000					540	!	
Hesperidin	mg		75											ID		
Phenolic compounds (see comment in legend)	mg			900					350					25	^^	
Pinus Epicatechins	mg			10					50					ID		
Procyanidolic Oligomers	mg			185		150				100		100		100		
Quercetin	mg		105						900					ID		
Resveratrol (3,4',5-trihydroxystilbene)	mg					400								ID		
Rutin	mg		25											ID		
Carotenoids																
Astaxanthin (marine carotenoid)	mg										3			ID		
beta Carotene	IU	4,500	15,000	11,250			15,000	6,250	15,000	17,500		12,500	15,000	13,750		ID
Carotenoids (mixed)	IU		0				5,000	6,250				542		5,625	***	ID
Lutein/Zeaxanthin	mg			6		6						4		5		
Lycopene	mg			15		20						2		15		
Glutathione Complex																
Acetyl-l-Cysteine	mg	90	300	50				no amt				63		76		ND
Cysteine	mg		75											ID		ND
Glutathione	mg	23		100						150		15		NR		ND

Table 3: Table of Recommended Daily Intakes *(Blended Standard) [continued]*

	Units													Standard		ND
Lipid Metabolism																
Acetyl-l-Carnitine	mg													500		ND
Carnitine	mg	450	300											500		ND
Choline	mg	360	500				150	750	55	138	500	150	55	94		3500 mg
Inositol	mg		125	200			50	63	55	63	500	200	55	125		ND
Lecithin	mg		125	250				200		63				350	*^	ND
alpha Linolenic Acid (an omega-3 essential fatty acid)	mg		350		750					2500		no amt		3,125		ND
Conjugated linoleic acid (CLA)	mg		no amt						6000		2500			ID		ND
Linoleic Acid (an omega-6 essential fatty acid)	mg			150					2000			no amt		ID		ND
gamma Linolenic Acid (GLA)	mg			25							300			ID	*^	ND
Omega-3 fish oil (EPA/ DHA)	mg							no amt		360	978	no amt		1,141		ND
Phosphatidylcholine	mg			200		3,350	1,304		300					ID		ND
Phosphatidylserine	mg			180										ID		ND
Minerals																
Boron	mg	300	5	3			2	3	4	3		3	2	3		20
Calcium	mg	225	1,750	800	1,100	1,250	1,000	600	750	350	100	1,150	500	800		2500 mg
Chromium (trivalent)	ug	1	275	200	120	160	200	300	300	300		250	300	238		ND
Copper	mg		3	1	1	2	2	3	2	3		2	2	2		10 mg
Fluorine (as fluoride)	mg				NR									ID		10 mg
Iodine	ug		163	100	NR		150		100	100		150	100	1,000	+	1100 ug
Iron	mg		NR	10		!!!	!!!	NR	23	15		NR	23	NR	**	45 mg
Magnesium	mg	75	875	600	100	500	500	525	375	400		650	375	[280]	!!	350 mg
Manganese	mg	18	7	6	2	4	20	10	13	4		5	13	7		11 mg
Molybdenum	ug	45	65	60	75		150		18	150		75	18	65		2000 ug
Potassium	mg		300	100			99		350	130			350	215		ND
Selenium	ug	180	150	250	128	175	200	38	150	150		200	150	150		400 ug
Silicon	mg			13					13	53		3	1	8		ND
Vanadium	ug	68	600					113	75			65	75	75		ND
Zinc	mg	36	40		15	23	40	13	30	28		25	23	25		40 mg
Other Nutritional Factors																
Arginine	mg					7,500								ID		ND
Betaine (trimethylglycine or TMG)	mg		no amt					no amt				350		350		ND
Bromelaine (digestive enzymes)	mg											no amt		ID		ND
Carnosine	mg						1,000							1,000		ND
Dimethylglycine (DMG)	mg					1,000				100				ID		ND
Dimethylaminoethanol (DMAE)	mg									100				ID		ND
Garlic extract (standardized)	mg					1,600								ID		ND
Gingko Biloba	mg							no amt			75			ID		ND
Glucosamine	mg			80				no amt						ID		ND
Glutamine	mg								1,500					ID		ND
Indole-3-Carbinol	mg					200					0.5 tsp			ID		ND
Lysine	mg		75											ID		ND
Melatonin	mg							2	3					ID		ND
Methionine	mg		75											ID		ND
Octacosanol	ug													ID		ND
Taurine	mg	675	300							50				ID		ND
Tyrosine	mg		500							50				ID		ND
Vinpocetine	mg													ID		ND

Notes for Table 3: Recommended Daily Intakes *(Blended Standard)*

Upper Limits (UL)

The upper level of intake considered safe for use by adults, incorporating a safety factor, as determined by the Food and Nutrition Board of the Institute of Medicine

References by author

Balch, PA. *Prescription for Nutritional Healing*, Avery Books, New York, NY, 2002.

Colgan, M. *Hormonal Health*, Apple Publishing, Vancouver, BC, 1996.

Mindell, E. *What You Should Know about Creating Your Personal Vitamin Plan*, Keats Pub., New Canaan, CT, 1996.

Murray, M and Pizzorno J. *Encyclopedia of Natural Medicine*, Prima Publishing, Rocklin, CA, 1998.

Murray, M. *Encyclopedia of Nutritional Supplements*, Prima Publishing, Rocklin, CA, 1996.

Passwater, RA. *The New Supernutrition*, Simon and Schuster Inc. New York, NY, 1991.

Strand, R. *What Your Doctor Doesn't Know about Nutritional Medicine May Be Killing You*, Thomas Nelson Inc. Nashville TN, 2002.

Whitaker, J. *Dr. Whitaker's Guide to Natural Healing*, Prima Publishing, Rocklin CA, 1996.

Perricone, N. *The Perricone Weight-loss Diet*, Ballantine Books, New York, 2005.

Kurzweil, R and Grossman, T. *Fantastic Voyage*, Holtzbrinck Publishers, 2004.

Atkins RC. *Dr. Atkins' Vita-nutrient Solution*, Fireside Printers, New York, 1999.

Miller, PL. and the Life Extension Foundation, *The Life Extension Revolution*, Bantam Dell, New York, 2005.

Higdon J. and the Linus Pauling Institute. *An Evidence-based Approach to Vitamins and Minerals*, Thieme Publishers, New York, 2003.

Legend

*	Colgan: lecithin specified in form of phosphatidyl-choline
**	Balch: only if an iron deficiency exists
***	Strand: conversion from mg to IU provided by Murray MT, *Encyclopedia of Nutritional Supplements*, page 25
^	Passwater: 1-2 caps estimated at 1000 mg/cap as lecithin
^^	Level of Phenolic Acids adapted from: Visioli F et al. *Atherosclerosis* 1995, 117: 25-32
^^^	Based on the recommended 2:1 ratio of alpha tocopherol to gamma tocopherol see Helzlsouer KJ et al, J Nat Canc Inst. 2000;92(24):2018-2023
!	Also includes values for hesperedin, quercetin, rutin, and pinus epicatechins
!!	350 mg represents the Upper Limit for a pharmacological agent only
!!!	pre-menopausal women only
†	Vitamin D and Iodine amounts adapted to reflect emerging science and/or changes to DRI amounts by Health Canada and the US Institute of Medicine. Safe Upper Limits also increased to reflect the new recommendations of the Food and Nutrition Board, Institute of Medicine
ID	Insufficient Data
NR	Not Recommended
[ ]	daily recommended intake truncated at 80% of Upper Safe Limit for that nutrient

continued from page 61

inclusion in the *Blended Standard*. These categories represent individuals who have poor-to-average diets, poor-to-average health, take little or no exercise and live a sedentary lifestyle, reflecting today's general profile of the North American adult population.

The recommendations for daily intake compiled in the *Blended Standard* prescribe appropriate levels of intake for each of the 18 Health Support criteria developed for the rating of each product. In turn, these 18 criteria are used to provide an overall product rating, represented on a five-star scale. Details of each criterion are discussed in Chapter Seven.

The *Table of Recommended Daily Intakes, shown* on pages 62-63, provides the daily nutritional recommendations of each authority, along with the median value for each nutrient incorporated into the *Blended Standard* derived from these recommendations.

Limitations of the Study

The products reviewed in this comparison represent the vast range of nutritional options available in the marketplace today. By necessity, NutriSearch has limited the selection to include only those products that meet specified criteria.

A qualifying product:

✓ must comprise a broad-spectrum nutritional supplement formulated for general preventive maintenance rather than a specified therapeutic use;

✓ must contain a comprehensive assortment of both minerals and vitamins;

✓ may contain assorted antioxidants and plant-based nutrients;

✓ must be formulated in tablet, capsule, powder, or liquid form and have a specified daily dosage; and

✓ must provide a comprehensive list of ingredients, along with specified amounts (in µg, mg or IU) for each nutrient in the formulation.

Individual products may contain nutrients other than those listed in the *Blended Standard*. With the exception of iron,* nutrients are *not* included in the comparison if those nutrients are not identified in the *Blended Standard*. In addition, while a manufacturer may list a nutrient identified in the *Blended Standard*, **the nutrient is not included in the comparison if the exact amount [microgram (µg), milligram (mg) or International Unit (IU)], of the nutrient is not provided or cannot be determined.** For example, if vitamin A in a product is shown as "5,000 IU of vitamin A with beta carotene" the entire amount is entered as

---

* *Due to findings on its potential toxicity, we have eliminated iron as a component of the Blended Standard; however, because of its continued use in many supplements, iron continues to be included in the criterion for potential toxicity.*

vitamin A because the precise amount of beta carotene cannot be determined.

Proprietary Blends

Some manufacturers list a collection of nutrients, usually those plant-based nutrients that comprise the flavonoids and polyphenols found in food-based sources, as a Proprietary Blend. **In such cases, where the specified amounts of the individual nutrients are not described on the label, it is not possible for NutriSearch to give credit for each nutrient in the blend.** Instead, NutriSearch will endeavour to provide credit for the major nutrient type only, if this can be determined from the labelling information, based on the milligram amounts of the general category as described on the label.

Manufacturing Quality

Our *initial* product rating does not consider compliance with current Good Manufacturing Practices (cGMP), nor does it reflect an analysis of product content. **The NutriSearch five-star rating is based solely on label claim.**

However, those manufacturers whose products achieve the maximum five-star rating are invited by *NutriSearch* to demonstrate their commitment to quality by providing proof of their level of GMP compliance and by furnishing a notarized certificate of analysis for their product(s). This requires submission of evidence of an independent audit of current manufacturing practices (GMP) and an independent laboratory analysis of product content, including identity, potency, and purity. Manufacturers who provide such standards of evidence qualify for the *NutriSearch Medals of Achievement Program.*™ Details of this program are discussed in Chapter Eight.

Qualifying the Products

All nutritional products considered for inclusion in this comparative guide are initially screened for excessive potency of specific nutrients, according to the Upper Limit of daily intake (UL) established by the US Food and Nutrition Board. The UL (shown in the right-hand column of the Table of Recommended Daily Intakes on pages 62-63) represents the upper level of intake for a specific nutrient deemed safe for use by adults.*

Any product containing three or more nutrients with potencies exceeding 150% of the Upper Limit is eliminated from further consideration. Disqualified products (if any) are listed in the Product Rating Tables with an appropriate notation.

---

* *The Food and Nutrition Board, Institute of Medicine, Washington, DC recently established the ULs for a number of vitamins and minerals. These values are shown in The Table of Recommended Daily Intakes, pages 62-63.*

The Final Product Rating (Star Rating)

Using the 18 Health Support criteria described in Chapter Seven, all qualifying products are evaluated using a series of algorithms (mathematical procedures) to arrive at a *Final Product Rating*. The development of each criterion is based on the scientific evidence available in the literature. Nutrient potencies are based on the median values of the pooled recommendations for intake established in the *Blended Standard*.

A five-star scale divided into half-star increments represents the *Final Product Rating*. A rating of five stars highlights those products possessing health support characteristics that are clearly superior to the majority of products on the market. Conversely, a rating of one star or less represents products possessing few, if any, of the health support characteristics reflected in the *Blended Standard*.

Due to significant differences in the regulatory environments of the differing countries reviewed in this guide, and the consequent impact of these regulations on allowable formulations, NutriSearch has found it necessary to adjust the final product ratings to accommodate these differences.

Consequently, a five-star rating for products in Colombia or Mexico may not equate to a five-star rating for products in Canada or the United States. The relative product ratings for each country must be considered only for products manufactured in the same country.

> *There are, in fact, two things:*
> *science and opinion.*
> *The former begets knowledge,*
> *the latter ignorance.*
>
> ~ *Hippocrates (460BC-377 BC)*

CHAPTER SEVEN:

PRODUCT RATING CRITERIA

This chapter explains the *Health Support Profile,* a set of mathematical models based on the 18 Health Support criteria described below. The *Health Support Profile* provides an overall ranking for each product included in this guide in accordance with the nutrient intake recommendations as described in the *Blended Standard.* Together, the NutriSearch *Blended Standard* and the 18 Health Support criteria form the basis of our analysis. For a detailed explanation of the *Blended Standard,* please refer to the previous chapter.

To evaluate a product, its rating for each Health Support criterion is calculated mathematically. This rating is determined by the nutrients and their potencies present in the product in relation to the requirements for each criterion.

Next, these 18 individual ratings for each product are pooled to provide a raw product score for that product. These scores represent a product's rating relative to all products evaluated within a particular market. Final product ratings are displayed as star ratings, shown in half-star increments from zero to five stars.

The five-star scale is, at once, both visual and intuitive: a five-star rating represents a product of the highest quality relative to all products evaluated in accordance with the *Health Support Profile* used in our analysis. Conversely, a one-star rating or less represents products possessing few, if any, of the characteristics for optimal nutrition as reflected in the *Blended Standard.*

The NutriSearch *Health Support Profile* is summarized in the following discussion. For a more detailed explanation of each criterion and the science supporting its development, the reader is referred to the *Comparative Guide to Nutritional Supplements,™ 5th (Professional) Edition* (available in English only). Information is also available on our website at *www. nutrisearch.ca.*

Health Support Profile

To receive a full point for any single Health Support criterion, the product must *meet or exceed* the benchmark established for that criterion. Each criterion uses a sliding scale, from 0% to 100%,

Completeness: looks to see if the product contains all the Blended Standard nutrients.

Potency: looks to see how much of each nutrient the product contains compared to the Blended Standard amounts.

Antioxidant Support: examines the nutrients that help to prevent or repair cellular damage caused by oxidation, including vitamin C, vitamin E, vitamin A, beta carotene, alpha-lipoic acid, lycopene, coenzyme Q10, iodine, and selenium

Immune Support: Recent scientific research confirms the vital roles that vitamin D and iodine play in maintaining our long-term health. This new criterion examines the many nutrients, including vitamin D and iodine, which help to ward off many of the most common degenerative diseases that shorten our lives.

Lipotropic Factors: examines those nutrients, including choline, lecithin, and inositol, that help remove toxins, including heavy metals like lead. The liver and the brain are two primary targets for the accumulation of fat-soluble toxins.

Ocular Health: Good eyesight and prevention of cataracts and macular degeneration require adequate levels of several nutrients, including vitamin C, vitamin E, vitamin A (including beta carotene), and the carotenoids, lutein and zeaxanthin.

Liver Health: examines those nutrients (including vitamin C, cysteine and n-acetyl cysteine, iodine, selenium, vitamin B2, and vitamin B3) that enhance liver function and optimize levels of glutathione, which helps cells to fight off toxic challenges.

Glycation Control: examines those nutrients (l-carnosine, alpha tocopherol, gamma tocopherol, vitamin C, and alpha-lipoic acid) that help slow the progress of many degenerative diseases, including Parkinson's disease, Alzheimer's disease, and cancer.

Metabolic Health: examines those nutrients that help the body handle its daily sugar load, keeping systems responsive to insulin and restoring lost insulin sensitivity. These nutrients include vitamin B3, vitamin B6, vitamin B12, vitamin C, vitamin D, vitamin E, biotin, coenzyme Q10, chromium, iodine, magnesium, manganese, and zinc.

Heart Health: examines nutrients that help protect the heart and cardiovascular system, including vitamin D, vitamin E, beta carotene, coenzyme Q10, calcium, iodine, magnesium, l-carnitine or acetyl-l-carnitine, procyanidolic oligomers (PCOs), phenolic compounds and lycopene.

Potential Toxicities: examines those nutrients that can build up in the body, possibly leading to toxic levels with long-term intake. This includes vitamin A and iron. Accidental overdose of iron-containing supplements is, in fact, a leading cause of fatal poisoning in children. Vitamin A is available, safely, as beta carotene, while adequate iron is easily obtainable for most people from foods.

Vitamin E Forms: While d-alpha tocopherol is the most common form of vitamin E, gamma tocopherol and other forms offer additional protection from inflammation, cancer, and other processes that can damage cells. High-dose supplementation with alpha tocopherol alone can reduce the level of gamma tocopherol in body tissues.

Mineral Forms: examines the molecules that minerals are bound with to help them cross into the bloodstream. Amino acid chelates and organic acid complexes (such as citrates and gluconates) mimic the natural mineral chelates that form during the digestive process. Chelated minerals also appear not to block other minerals from being absorbed, unlike many of the less expensive mineral salts (carbonates, sulphates, and chlorides).

Methylation Support: looks at those nutrients, including vitamin B2, vitamin B6, vitamin B12, folic acid, and trimethylglycine, required for the body to produce methyl donor molecules. Methyl donors help reduce homocysteine levels in the blood, protecting the arteries and nerve fibres.

Bone Health: examines the nutrients that assist in bone remodeling, vital to ward off osteoporosis and other diseases that weaken the skeletal framework. These nutrients include vitamin D, vitamin K, vitamin C, vitamin B6, vitamin B12, folic acid, boron, calcium, magnesium, silicon, and zinc.

Inflammation Control: examines the nutrients responsible for reducing inflammation at the cellular level, such as omega-3 oils—including those found in fish oil (eicosapentaenoic and docosahexaenoic acids, or EPA and DHA)—linolenic acid, gamma tocopherol, alpha-lipoic acid, vitamin C, vitamin D, iodine, flavonoids, procyanidolic oligomers (PCOs), and the phenolic compounds. Chronic inflammation can lead to serious degenerative disease, including heart disease, cancers, and arthritis.

Phenolic Compounds Profile: examines a specific group of phenolic compounds (polyphenolic acids and their derivatives), known to be exceptionally potent defenders against free radicals. Phenols derived from olives, green tea, and curcumin are also known to improve major risk factors for cardiovascular disease, including lowering the impact of inflammation.

Bioflavonoid Profile: examines the bioflavonoid family of nutrients, which work throughout the body to attack free radicals and support many bodily fuctions. These important nutrients include citrus flavonoids, soy isoflavones, quercetin, quercitrin, hesperidin, rutin, bilberry, assorted berry extracts, and PCOs (including resveratrol, grape seed, and pine bark extracts).

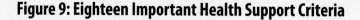

Figure 9: Eighteen Important Health Support Criteria

where partial points are awarded for the partial fulfilment of the criterion. The last criterion, *Potential Toxicities,* penalizes the product if the formulation exceeds defined limits of daily intake for those nutrients (vitamin A and iron) that demonstrate potential cumulative toxicities.

For each criterion, we address the fundamental question posed; in turn, each question presents the logical argument that forms the basis of our mathematical model for that criterion.

1. Completeness

The human body requires several vitamins and vitamin-like substances, a diverse group of plant-based antioxidants, numerous trace elements and minerals, and several essential fatty acids. Most of these substances can only be obtained through the diet. In all, 47 nutrients and nutrient categories comprise our *Blended Standard*—the benchmark upon which our analysis is built. This criterion assesses whether the product contains all of the *Blended Standard* nutrients.

Does the product contain the full spectrum of nutrients and nutrient categories listed in the Blended Standard and considered essential for optimal health? To qualify, a nutrient or nutrient category must be present at a dosage that is at least 20% of the value in the Blended Standard.

2. Potency

The potencies for the 47 essential nutrients and nutrient categories used in our *Blended Standard* reflect the need for supplementation with some nutrients at levels considerably higher than their recommended dietary intakes. This criterion assesses how much of each nutrient the product contains compared to the *Blended Standard.*

For each nutrient in the product, what is the level of potency relative to the potency for that nutrient in the Blended Standard?

3. Mineral Forms

Minerals are essential components of our cells and serve as cofactors in the thousands of chemical reactions that power the machinery of the cell. Throughout the body, minerals also form critical structural components, regulate the action of nerves and muscles, maintain the cell's water balance, and control the acidity of the cell and extracellular fluids. While minerals comprise only 4% to 5% of our total body weight, life would not be possible without them. This criterion examines the various mineral forms that differentially affect the ability of the minerals to be absorbed into the blood, making them available to our cells.

For those minerals included in a formulation, how many are found in their most bioavailable forms as amino acid chelates or organic acid complexes?

4. *Vitamin E Forms*

Vitamin E comes in many different forms, each of which has important benefits in cellular function. In its natural form, the most common type of vitamin E is *d*-alpha tocopherol; synthetic vitamin E, which is most commonly found in supplements as *d/l*-alpha tocopherol, is only half as effective as the natural form. Another form of vitamin E, gamma tocopherol, possesses distinctive chemical properties that differentiate it from alpha tocopherol. Studies show that gamma tocopherol reduces chronic inflammation and protects against cancers of the colon and prostate better than alpha tocopherol. This criterion assesses the product for the various forms of vitamin E and their bioactivity.

Does the product contain the natural (d) isomer of alpha tocopherol or does the product contain the less useful synthetic form of alpha tocopherol? Does the product contain gamma tocopherol (or a mixture of gamma, beta, and delta tocopherols) at a potency of up to one half the potency of alpha tocopherol in the same product? What is the potency of gamma tocopherol or mixed tocopherols in the product, compared to the potency for gamma tocopherol in the Blended Standard?

5. *Immune Support*

An explosion of research over the past decade has uncovered vitamin D as a vital component to our immune systems. Working in conjunction with other micronutrients, vitamin D can help protect us against many of the most common degenerative diseases, including heart disease, stroke, cancer, multiple sclerosis, dementia, and many others.

Another nutrient recently discovered as vital to immune support is iodine. The high iodine concentration of the thymus gland is evidence of the important role played by iodine in the immune system—a role likely related to the element's antioxidant powers.

Many other nutrients, including vitamin A, vitamin C, vitamin E, zinc, selenium, and the B-vitamins B_1, B_2, B_5 (pantothenic acid), B_6, B_{12}, and folic acid, are also indispensable to a healthy immune system. This criterion assesses the product for vitamin D and iodine levels and for the presence of these other nutrients that boost the immune response.

Does the product contain vitamin D and iodine at the potencies described in the Blended Standard? Does the product also contain beta carotene and vitamin A, vitamin C, vitamin E, zinc, selenium, and the B-vitamins B_1, B_2, B_5 (pantothenic acid), B_6, B_{12}, and folic acid at the potencies established in the Blended Standard?

6. *Antioxidant Support*

The weight of scientific evidence supports supplementation with antioxidants in the prevention and treatment of many of today's common ailments. As was anticipated decades ago by leading researchers, high-dose supplementation with antioxidants has gained a significant role in the prevention and treatment of many of today's common ailments. However, antioxidants do not work in isolation. For this reason, it is vital to supplement with a wide spectrum of antioxidants—an approach that is reflective of what occurs in nature. This criterion examines the nutrients that help to prevent or repair cellular damage caused by oxidation.

Does the product contain vitamin C, vitamin E (including alpha tocopherol and gamma [or mixed] tocopherols), vitamin A, beta carotene, alpha lipoic acid, lycopene, coenzyme Q10, selenium, and iodine at potencies up to 100% of the potencies for these nutrients in the Blended Standard?

7. *Bone Health*

As living tissue, healthy bones require at least 24 bone-building materials, including several vitamins, minerals, trace elements, and protein. The most important minerals are calcium, magnesium, phosphorus, and potassium; equally important is the balance between these minerals. This criterion examines the nutrients in a product that assist in bone remodelling, a process vital in warding off osteoporosis and other diseases that weaken the skeletal framework.

Does the product contain vitamin D, vitamin K, vitamin C, vitamin B$_6$, vitamin B$_{12}$, folic acid, boron, calcium, magnesium, silicon, and zinc at potencies up to 100% of the potencies for these nutrients in the Blended Standard?

8. *Heart Health*

Individuals with high dietary intakes of antioxidant vitamins, certain minerals, and several plant-based compounds exhibit a lower-than-average risk of cardiovascular disease. This criterion examines several nutrients, including the recently discovered cardioprotective powerhouses, iodine and vitamin D, that are known to benefit the heart and cardiovascular system by reducing oxidative stress and suppressing inflammation.

Does the product contain vitamin D, iodine, vitamin E (including alpha tocopherol and gamma [or mixed] tocopherols), beta carotene, coenzyme Q10, calcium, magnesium, carnitine or acetyl-l-carnitine, procyanidolic oligomers (PCOs), phenolic compounds, and lycopene at potencies up to 100% of the potencies for those nutrients and nutrient categories in the Blended Standard?

9. *Liver Health (detoxification)*

Glutathione is a water-phase anti-oxidant and one of three vital free radical–scavenging mechanisms in the cell. Glutathione status is a sensitive indicator of cellular health and of the cell's ability to resist toxic challenges. It is also the liver's foremost detoxifying agent. While dietary glutathione is efficiently absorbed in the gut, the same is not the case for nutritional supplementation.

Iodine is another important nutrient for liver health and detoxification. Iodine's ability to lessen the potential damage of hydrogen peroxide provides support for the work of the glutathione peroxidase enzyme system in helping to remove toxic agents from the body. This criterion examines those nutrients that optimize levels of glutathione and enhance liver function.

Does the product contain iodine, vitamin C, n-acetyl-cysteine (including cysteine), selenium, vitamin B_2, and vitamin B_3 (including niacin and niacinamide), at potencies up to 100% of the potencies for these nutrients in the Blended Standard?

10. *Metabolic Health (glucose control)*

Diabetes is a chronic disorder of carbohydrate, fat, and protein metabolism. The disease begins as a constellation of metabolic changes associated with chronically high insulin levels and elevated blood-sugar levels, a condition known as *Insulin Resistance.* The development of insulin resistance is multifactorial; however, complications associated with this prediabetic disorder can be resolved effectively through conscientious dietary and lifestyle changes, including supplementation with several vitamins and minerals essential for metabolic support and the close regulation of glucose metabolism. This criterion examines those nutrients that help the body handle its daily sugar load, keeping systems responsive to insulin and restoring lost insulin sensitivity.

Does the product contain vitamin B_3 (including niacin and niacinamide), vitamin B_6, vitamin B_{12}, vitamin C, vitamin E (including alpha tocopherol and gamma [or mixed] tocopherols), vitamin D, iodine, biotin, coenzyme Q_{10}, chromium, magnesium, manganese, and zinc at potencies up to 100% of the potencies for these nutrients in the Blended Standard?

11. *Ocular Health*

Good eyesight and the prevention of cataracts and macular degeneration require adequate levels of several nutrients known to reduce the level of oxidative stress in the retina and lens of the eye.

Does the product contain the antioxidants, vitamin C, vitamin E (including alpha and gamma [or mixed] tocopherols), vitamin A (including beta carotene), and the carotenoids lutein and zeaxanthin at potencies up to 100% of the potencies for these nutrients in the Blended Standard?

12. *Methylation Support*

Over 40 major clinical studies confirm that high homocysteine levels are a predictive marker for heart disease, stroke, and peripheral artery disease. In fact, up to 40% of patients with heart disease express elevated levels of homocysteine. Deficiencies in certain B-complex vitamins are known to increase circulating levels of homocysteine; conversely, supplementation with these nutrients can significantly reduce circulating homocysteine by converting it to harmless methionine and cysteine. This criterion looks at those nutrients required for the body to reduce homocysteine levels in the blood.

Does the product contain vitamin B_2, vitamin B_6, vitamin B_{12}, folic acid, and trimethylglycine at potencies up to 100% of the potencies for these nutrients in the Blended Standard?

13. *Lipotropic Factors*

The liver and the brain are two primary targets for the accumulation of fat-soluble toxins, including pesticides and heavy metals (such as lead). Within the liver, choline and inositol assist with the elimination and removal of these noxious compounds through their ability to mobilize fats and bile. Known as *lipotropic* (fat-moving) factors, these agents have a long history of use within the naturopathic community, helping to restore and enhance liver function and treat a number of common liver ailments. This criterion examines those lipotropic agents that help the liver mobilize fat stores and remove toxins.

Does the product contain the important lipotropic factors choline, or lecithin (phosphatidylcholine), and inositol at potencies up to 100% of the potencies for these nutrients in the Blended Standard?

14. *Inflammation Control*

Chronic inflammation is a principal mechanism by which degenerative disease takes root. Changing the balance within the body to favour the production of anti-inflammatory chemical messengers and lower the levels of inflammation is therefore an important preventive measure. This criterion examines the nutrients responsible for reducing inflammation at the cellular level, such as the omega 3 oils—particularly those found in fish and flaxseed oils.

Recent evidence shows that Vitamin D also expresses potent anti-inflammatory actions. The hormone activates several genes controlling the manufacture of inflammation-suppressing chemicals produced in specialized white blood cells, which dampen the over-response of the immune system common in allergic reactions. As well, iodine—likely in its molecular form—exhibits anti-inflammatory and antiproliferative activities that are important factors in determining cardiovascular health, and in reducing the risk of inflammatory cancers of the breast, stomach, endometrium, and ovaries.

Does the product contain eicosapentaenoic and docosahexaenoic acids, linolenic acid, gamma tocopherol, alpha lipoic acid, vitamin C, vitamin D, iodine, flavonoids, procyanidolic oligomers, and the phenolic compounds from green tea, olive, and turmeric extracts, at potencies up to 100% of the potencies for these nutrients or nutrient categories in the Blended Standard?

15. Glycation Control

Aging—the outcome of the conflict between chemistry and biology in living systems—introduces chronic cumulative chemical changes that compromise the structure and function of important biomolecules within our cells. We now know that changes to these molecular structures, driven by unrelenting oxidative stress, can render them dysfunctional. Their accumulation, the detritus of an ongoing oxidative war within the cell, is a hallmark of the aging process. This criterion examines those nutrients that help slow the progress of glycation.

Does the product contain l-carnosine, vitamin E (including alpha tocopherol

and gamma [or mixed] tocopherols), vitamin C, and alpha lipoic acid at potencies up to 100% of the potencies for those nutrients or nutrient categories listed in the Blended Standard?

16. Bioflavonoid Profile

The flavonoids are known as nature's biological response modifiers because of their ability to alter the body's reactions to allergens, viruses, and carcinogens, and to protect cellular tissues against oxidative attack. Flavonoids, a group of highly coloured pigments found in the edible pulp of many fruits and vegetables, impart a bitter taste when isolated. Citrus fruits, such as oranges, lemons, limes, grapefruit, and kiwi, are particularly rich sources of flavonoids. This criterion examines the bioflavonoid family of nutrients, which works throughout the body to attack free radicals, suppress inflammation, and support cellular functions.

Does the product contain a mixture of bioflavonoids (including citrus and other flavonoids, bilberry and related extracts, hesperidin, quercetin, quercitrin, rutin, soy, silymarin, and related milk thistle extracts), and PCOs (including grape seed and grape seed extract, Hawthorne berry and Hawthorne berry extract, pine bark and pine bark extract, pycnogenol and resveratrol) at potencies up to 100% of the recommended potencies for mixed bioflavonoids and PCOs in the Blended Standard?

17. *Phenolic Compounds Profile*

The scientific evidence supporting the health benefits of polyphenols is strong. They are powerful free radical antagonists, recognized for their ability to reduce cardiovascular disease and cancer, and they demonstrate potent anti-inflammatory, antiviral, antibacterial, antiallergic, antihaemorrhagic, and immune-enhancing properties. The most intensely studied of the phenolic compounds include those isolated from: turmeric, a perennial herb of the ginger family and a major ingredient in curry; green tea, a rich source of compounds called catechins; and extracts from the fruit of the olive tree. This criterion examines these specific phenolic compounds, all of them known to be exceptionally potent free radical antagonists.

Does the product contain phenolic compounds (polyphenolic acids and their derivatives), including cinnamon bark and cinnamon bark extract, cranberry and cranberry extract, curcumin, fenugreek, ginger and gingerols, green tea leaf and green tea extracts, olive fruit and olive extracts, papaya, pomegranate fruit and pomegranate extract, rosemary, and turmeric rhizome, at the potency for this nutrient category established in the Blended Standard?

18. *Potential Toxicities*

In order to optimize its preventive benefits, the strategy of nutritional supplementation is to encourage long-term use. Consequently, there exists a potential risk for consumers with regard to the cumulative toxicity of particular nutrients. Most nutrients used in nutritional supplements have a high degree of safety; however, some nutrients require a degree of prudence when it comes to long-term use. Both iron and vitamin A (retinol) can become toxic when taken in high doses over a long period. Accidental overdose of iron-containing supplements is, in fact, a leading cause of fatal poisoning in children, and too much vitamin A during pregnancy can cause birth defects. Vitamin A is available, safely, as beta carotene, while adequate iron is easily obtained, for most people, from a variety of foods. This criterion examines the levels of preformed vitamin A (retinol) and iron in the product and penalizes the product rating if it contains too much of either nutrient.

Does the nutritional supplement contain vitamin A and iron? Does the potency of vitamin A exceed 100% of the potency for that nutrient in the Blended Standard? Does the potency of iron exceed 5 mg/day?

Summary

The 18 individual Health Support ratings, as described above, are pooled for each product to provide a raw product score. These scores are then separated statistically to present a product's rating relative to all products evaluated. Final product ratings are displayed as star ratings, shown in half-star increments from zero to five stars. The five-star scale is, at once, both visual and intuitive: a five-star product represents a product of the highest quality relative to all products evaluated in accordance with the comprehensive NutriSearch *Health Support Profile* used in our analysis. Conversely, a one-star rating or less represents products possessing few, if any, of the characteristics for optimal nutrition as reflected in the NutriSearch *Blended Standard*.

**Quality means doing it right
when no one is looking.**

~ Henry Ford (1863 – 1947)

CHAPTER EIGHT:

MEDALS OF ACHIEVEMENT

Whether talking about drugs or nutritional supplements, the use of accepted standards of manufacturing (GMP) and laboratory verification of the finished product are the consumer's only real assurance of quality and safety. These assurances are provided by federal regulations that govern the manufacture and sale of all natural health products—regulations that can differ markedly from country to country.

Canada and the United States

The Government of Canada requires that all manufacturers of nutritional supplements sold in or into Canada comply with federally mandated manufacturing and quality standards developed specifically for natural health products (NHPs). While considerably more stringent than Canada's regulations for foods, the regulations for NHPs do not match the level of oversight required for pharmaceutical products. The regulations require the manufacturer to obtain the requisite site and product licenses prior to selling any

natural health product in Canada. Health Canada is empowered to conduct post-market product audits; however, these regulations are lacking in enforcement. It is common for facilities to have a valid site license without undergoing an actual audit of either plant or finished product. Canada's regulations are not as rigorous as the requirements in Australia, where natural health products are treated as listed medicines and must meet stringent pharmaceutical-grade requirements prior to marketing (including ongoing physical post-market product audits). Nevertheless, Canada's regulatory environment provides a reasonable level of quality and safety.

On June 25, 2007, the US Food and Drug Authority (FDA) established regulations entitled *Current Good Manufacturing Practice (cGMP) In Manufacturing, Packaging, Labeling, Or Holding Operations For Dietary Supplements*. These regulations compel companies who manufacture, package, label, or hold a dietary supplement to follow established good manufacturing practices (cGMP) to ensure the quality of the dietary supplements manufactured. The regulations, which were phased in over the last several years are now in effect.

While a step in the right direction, the new US regulations continue to be based on modified food-grade standards, rather than modelled after more stringent pharmaceutical-grade GMPs. Consequently, products manufactured in the United States do not approach the standards of evidence or oversight required for products manufactured in either Canada or Australia. The FDA does not require manufacturers to register their products or obtain licensing approval before manufacturing or selling dietary supplements. Similarly, it is up to the manufacturer, not any government agency, to determine if their nutritional products are safe. The FDA only investigates products *after* problems are found, usually through reports of adverse reactions.

Both the United States and Canada fail to pass muster when it comes to ongoing post-market surveillance of product quality. While empowered to do so, neither country actively pursues post-market product audits requiring laboratory evaluation of product identity, potency, and safety. Because of this, the purchase of nutritional supplements in both the United States and Canada continues to remain an issue of "buyer beware."

Latin America

Throughout Latin America, dietary supplements are commonly registered as prescription drugs, over-the-counter (OTC) drugs, or food supplements and are subject to diverse regulations dependent on the country of sale. The differentiation between the terms 'food' and 'drug' is important due to the varying levels of regulatory oversight and differences in the requirements for GMP between these categories.

In Mexico, nutritional supplements are generally regulated as foods and, while submission of ingredient lists and labelling information is necessary, there is no requirement for site or product licensing prior to marketing a product. There is no post-market surveillance for ongoing GMP compliance; neither is there any post-market product audit requiring laboratory verification of product identity, potency, and safety. Higher quality nutritional supplements containing nutrients whose potencies exceed those prescribed in the regulations must be registered in Mexico as medicinal products; these products are subject to more stringent regulations that govern pharmaceutical products.

In Colombia, supplements are regulated under a category that is separate from either foods or medicines, and dietary supplements are required to be registered prior to market approval. Like Canada, their manufacture requires GMPs that fall between foods and pharmaceuticals, providing a higher level of safety for the consumer. Products sold in or into Colombia are regularly scrutinized by label claim; however, there is no requirement for post-market product audits necessitating laboratory evaluation of product identity, potency, and safety.

In both Mexico and Colombia ingredients other than vitamins and minerals are permitted for use in nutritional supplements; however, the types of ingredients permitted can vary between countries. Ginseng, for example, is permitted as a botanical herb in Colombia, but not in Mexico, where ginseng is regarded as an ingredient with a pharmacological action and falls under the category of a registered medicine.

Another challenge faced by supplement manufacturers selling in or into Latin American countries, such as Mexico and Colombia, is the variance in allowable potencies of nutrients in a given formulation. This may require a North American manufacturer to extensively modify a formulation in order to legally sell into these countries.

Such regulatory differences pose a particular conundrum for NutriSearch when reviewing the products of these countries, as the same product from a given manufacturer may have significantly different formulations and nutrient potencies. Such products will, consequently, be rated differently (according to our established criteria) depending on the country of sale for that product.

For this reason, we caution the reader that our NutriSearch product rating for any given product must be viewed _only_ within the context of how that product compares to other products within the same jurisdiction. That is, the rating for a product manufactured for Mexico or Colombia may not be equivalent to the rating given to that same product manufactured for Canada or the United States.

Assessing Product Quality

How a nutritional product is made—what's in it and what's not supposed to be in it—is critical to the quality and safety of the finished product. Unless a product is manufactured to a standard of quality that is based on acceptable good manufacturing practices (GMP) and unless that finished product is audited regularly through independent laboratory testing, the consumer cannot be certain that _what is on the label is actually in the bottle._

That is why NutriSearch has introduced a level of product assessment, called the _NutriSearch Medals of Achievement Program,_ ™ that goes beyond assessment of product content and investigates how a product is manufactured (level of GMP compliance). Through independent laboratory testing, we also investigate what is actually in the finished product.

This higher standard of evidence incurs considerable cost and effort on the part of the selected manufacturers; consequently, we have offered it only to those manufacturers whose products merit a five-star rating based on our initial analysis. The assessment is entirely voluntary and the expense for GMP audits and laboratory testing is borne by each individual manufacturer.

Products that achieve a five-star Final Product Rating are eligible to participate in the *NutriSearch Medals of Achievement Program*, which awards GOLD medals based on an assessment of the level of GMP and on independent laboratory verification of the product's formulation.

Certification and Analysis Programs

Currently, there are two independent non-government programs available in North America and elsewhere for the evaluation of manufacturing standards for nutritional supplements:

✓ NSF International Dietary Supplement Verification Program

✓ United States Pharmacopeial (USP) Dietary Supplement Verification Program

NutriSearch accepts certification from either of these programs as evidence of a manufacturer's level of GMP compliance. NutriSearch also accepts certification by Health Canada's Natural Health Products Directorate (NHPD) and Australia's Therapeutic Goods Administration (TGA) as evidence of compliance with nutraceutical-to-pharmaceutical level GMPs.

Evaluation of the contents of the product is a second requirement for those manufacturers seeking the NutriSearch GOLD Medal status as a Top-Rated product. For this, NutriSearch accepts the results of product analyses conducted by the NSF International Dietary Supplement Verification Program and the USP Dietary Supplement Verification Program as acceptable standards of evidence. To qualify for Gold Medal status, a company must submit its finished product to either of these testing agencies for a complete analysis of content, including identity, potency, and safety. A notarized certificate of analysis of the active ingredients of the finished product must accompany notarized proof of GMP compliance.

Previously, NutriSearch recognized Certificates of Analysis provided by independent laboratories certified by the International Standards Organization (ISO) as acceptable standards of evidence. This option has now been terminated due to recent public disclosures of the widespread practice of 'dry labbing' within the nutritional industry (while ISO certifies a testing lab, the organization does not conduct any ongoing performance audits).

Dry labbing is the unethical and fraudulent practice of manufacturing test results to meet a manufacturer's written specifications without actually conducting any laboratory evaluation of that product. If you wish to learn more about this serious misrepresentation of product quality—common throughout the US supplement industry—please view the following *Dateline NBC* exposé posted on YouTube: http://www.youtube.com/playlist?list=PL60B2472EB8543527

Summary

Together, evidence of GMP certification *and* proof of product content are essential to demonstrate that a product meets recognized standards of evidence for manufacturing quality. Most importantly, it is the consumer's only real assurance that *what is on the label is actually in the bottle.*

For a complete description of our *NutriSearch Medals of Achievement* *Program*, please refer to the *NutriSearch Comparative Guide to Nutritional Supplements, 5th (Professional) Edition* (available in English only). Information is also available on our website at *www. nutrisearch.ca.*

> **I have the simplest tastes.**
> **I am always satisfied with the best.**
>
> *~ Oscar Wilde (1854 - 1900)*

CHAPTER NINE:

TOP-RATED PRODUCTS

In this inaugural edition of the *NutriSearch Comparative Guide for the Americas*, we provide you with a close-up look at the Leading Vitamin Manufacturers by Market Share, as organized by country and as identified by global market research company Euromonitor International.

For each of the leading national manufacturers listed by Euromonitor, we have selected the highest rated broad-spectrum nutritional product that we have identified through our field research. Each product is analyzed using our *Blended Standard* and 18 *Health Support* Criteria, then rated according to the five-star model established for that country. In some cases, and despite our best efforts, where we have been unable to identify a qualifying product of a leading manufacturer, we have duly noted this in the accompanying tables (please refer to pages 66 and 67 for our qualifying criteria).

These products are graphically portrayed, allowing you to visually examine how each product performs in relation to our 18 *Health Support* criteria. These criteria are shown in the legend. Each graph displays the product name,

along with the product's overall rating in that country. Ratings are indicated on a scale of five stars, in half-star increments.

Where a particular manufacturer markets gender-specific products, both the men's and women's products are shown, if possible. Where a *NutriSearch Gold Medal of Achievement* has been earned, the five stars shown in the product graph are depicted in gold, and the medal is superimposed on the graph.

After reviewing each region, one company stood above all others; NutriSearch has selected a single product from this company that we believe provides exceptional value for three reasons:

✓ The product's overall rating in each country;

✓ The product's qualification as a NutriSearch GOLD Medal recipient in each country; and

✓ the public and scientific reputation of the company behind the product.

In the considered opinion of NutriSearch, this product represents the 'Best of the Best' and is identified as our *Editor's Choice.*

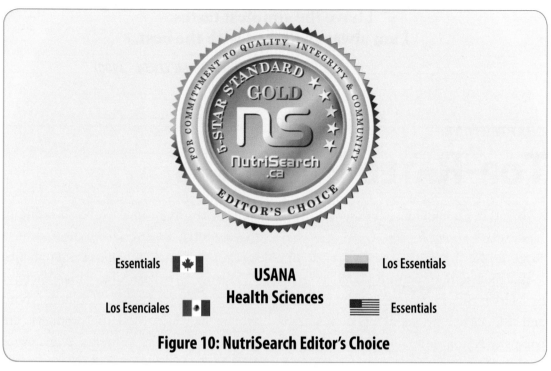

Essentials 🇨🇦　　USANA　Los Essentials
Los Esenciales 🇲🇽　Health Sciences　Essentials

Figure 10: NutriSearch Editor's Choice

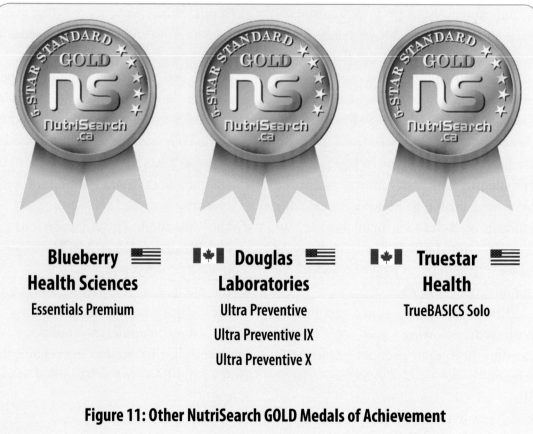

Blueberry 🇺🇸　🇨🇦 **Douglas** 🇺🇸　🇨🇦 **Truestar**
Health Sciences　**Laboratories**　**Health**

Essentials Premium　Ultra Preventive　TrueBASICS Solo

Ultra Preventive IX

Ultra Preventive X

Figure 11: Other NutriSearch GOLD Medals of Achievement

Table 4: 🇨🇦 Canadian Leading Manufacturers by Market Share

Manufacturer Name	Market Share	Top-Rated Product for this Manufacturer	Star Rating
Jamieson Laboratories Ltd	28.8%	Jamieson Mega-Vim	★★★☆☆
Pfizer Inc	15.6%	Centrum Advantage	★★☆☆☆
Amway Corp	2.4%	Nutrilite Daily Free	★★⯪☆☆
Valeant Pharmaceuticals International Inc	2.3%	~ No Qualifying Product Found ~	
WN Pharmaceuticals Ltd	1.4%	Webber Naturals Multisure Men 50+	★★★★⯪
		Webber Naturals Multisure Women 50+	★★★★⯪
Bayer AG	1.0%	One-a-Day WeightSmart	★★⯪☆☆
Otsuka Holdings Co Ltd	0.9%	Nature Made Multi for Her 50+	★★⯪☆☆
		Nature Made Multi for Him 50+	★★☆☆☆
Herbalife Ltd	0.5%	Herbalife Multivitamin Complex	★★☆☆☆
USANA Health Sciences Inc	0.5%	USANA Essentials	★★★★★
Nu Skin Enterprises Inc	0.4%	Pharmanex Vitox	★★★⯪☆

Data From Euromonitor Passport, Brand Shares: Vitamins
© 2013 Euromonitor International, a market research company. www.euromonitor.com

Table 5: 🇨🇴 Colombian Leading Manufacturers by Market Share

Manufacturer Name	Market Share	Top-Rated Product for this Manufacturer	Star Rating
Pfizer Inc	21.4%	Centrum Silver	★★⯪☆☆
Tecnoquímicas SA	15.7%	McK Vitafull Senior	★★☆☆☆
JGB SA, Laboratorios	7.2%	JGB Tarrito Rojo	★☆☆☆☆
Omnilife SA de CV, Grupo	6.0%	Omnilife Omni Plus	★☆☆☆☆
GlaxoSmithKline Plc	4.2%	~ No Qualifying Product Found ~	
Merck KGaA	3.8%	Cebio Forte	★★⯪☆☆
Bayer AG	2.7%	Natale Easy	⯪☆☆☆☆
Procaps SA, Laboratorios	1.8%	Procaps Multivit M	⯪☆☆☆☆
4Life Research USA LLC	1.8%	4Life Transfer Factor B C V	⯪☆☆☆☆
Laboratorios La Santé SA	1.2%	~ No Qualifying Product Found ~	

Data From Euromonitor Passport, Brand Shares: Vitamins
© 2013 Euromonitor International, a market research company. www.euromonitor.com

Table 6: 🇲🇽 Méxican Leading Manufacturers by Market Share

Manufacturer Name	Market Share	Top-Rated Product for this Manufacturer	Star Rating
Herbalife Ltd	21.9%	Herbalife Número 2	★☆☆☆☆
Farmacias Similares SA de CV	10.7%	Simi Vitaminas	⯪☆☆☆☆
Boehringer Ingelheim GmbH	7.2%	Pharmaton Protect	★☆☆☆☆
Bayer AG	5.1%	Berocca Vitaminas, Calcio y Magnesio	⯪☆☆☆☆
Pfizer Inc	5.1%	Centrum Silver	★⯪☆☆☆
Sanofi	4.4%	*~ No Qualifying Product Found ~*	
Omnilife SA de CV, Grupo	4.3%	Omnilife OmniPlus Supreme	★☆☆☆☆
Merck & Co Inc	3.7%	*~ No Qualifying Product Found ~*	
Valeant Pharmaceuticals International Inc	2.1%	Bedoyecta Complejo B con ácido fólico	★☆☆☆☆
Merck KGaA	2.0%	*~ No Qualifying Product Found ~*	
Bomuca SA de CV	1.6%	Vivioptal Cápsulas	★☆☆☆☆
USANA Health Sciences Inc	1.5%	Los Esenciales de USANA	★★★★★
Amway Corp	1.3%	Nutrilite Double X	⯪☆☆☆☆
General Nutrition Centers Inc	0.4%	GNC TR Ultra Mega	★★★⯪☆
Representaciones e Investigaciones Médicas SA de CV (RIMSA)	0.4%	Rimsa Vitalen Complejo B	⯪☆☆☆☆
Laboratorios Silanes SA de CV	0.4%	*~ No Qualifying Product Found ~*	
Banner Pharmacaps Inc	0.4%	*~ No Qualifying Product Found ~*	
Abbott Laboratories Inc	0.3%	Ensure	★☆☆☆☆
Bristol-Myers Squibb Co	0.2%	*~ No Qualifying Product Found ~*	
Productos Medix SA de CV	0.2%	*~ No Qualifying Product Found ~*	

Data From Euromonitor Passport, Brand Shares: Vitamins
© 2013 Euromonitor International, a market research company. www.euromonitor.com

Table 7: 🇺🇸 United States Leading Manufacturers by Market Share

Manufacturer Name	Market Share	Top-Rated Product for this Manufacturer	Star Rating
NBTY Inc	6.9%	Solgar Male Multiple	★★★★½
		Solgar Female Multiple	★★★★
Otsuka Holdings Co Ltd	5.6%	Nature Made Multi for Her 50+	★½
		Nature Made Multi for Him 50+	★★
Pfizer Inc	3.8%	Centrum Silver Men	★½
		Centrum Silver Women	★½
General Nutrition Centers Inc	3.5%	GNC Mega Men Liquid	★★★★
		~ No Similar Women's Product ~	
Dr Willmar Schwabe GmbH & Co KG	2.8%	~ No Qualifying Product Found ~	
Bayer AG	2.6%	One-a-Day Men's 50+ Advantage	★½
		One-a-Day Women's 50+ Advantage	★½
Atrium Innovations Inc	2.2%	Douglas Laboratories Ultra Preventive X	☆☆☆☆☆
Herbalife Ltd	1.6%	Herbalife Multivitamin Complex	★★
Shaklee Corp	1.5%	Shaklee Vita-Lea Gold Vitamin K	★★★½
Amway Corp	1.5%	Nutrilite Daily Free	★½
Church & Dwight Co Inc	1.2%	VitaFusion MultiVites	★½
Forever Living Products International, LLC	1.2%	~ No Qualifying Product Found ~	
Nature's Sunshine Products Inc	1.1%	Nature's Sunshine Super Supplemental	★★★
Melaleuca Inc	1.0%	Melaleuca Vitality Men's	★★★½
		Melaleuca Vitality Women's	★★
IdeaSphere Inc	1.0%	Allergy Research Group Steady On Powder	★★★★½
Plethico Pharmaceuticals Ltd	0.8%	Natrol My Favorite Multiple Iron Free	★★★★½
Reckitt Benckiser Plc (RB)	0.8%	~ No Qualifying Product Found ~	
USANA Health Sciences Inc	0.7%	USANA Essentials	☆☆☆☆☆
Nutraceutical Corp	0.5%	KAL Enhanced Energy Supreme Iron Free	★★★★½
Life Extension Foundation Inc	0.5%	Life Extension Mix	★★★★★
Sunrider International Inc	0.4%	~ No Qualifying Product Found ~	
Nu Skin Enterprises Inc	0.3%	Pharmanex Vitox	★★★½
Unicity International Inc	0.3%	Unicity Core Health Basics	★½

Manufacturer Name	Market Share	Top-Rated Product for this Manufacturer	Star Rating
Walgreen Co	0.1%	Walgreens A thru Z Select Ultimate Men's	★⯨
		Walgreens A thru Z Select Ultimate Women's	★⯨

Data From Euromonitor Passport, Brand Shares: Vitamins
© 2013 Euromonitor International, a market research company. www.euromonitor.com

Health Support Graph Legend

1. Completeness
2. Potency
3. Mineral Forms
4. Vitamin E Forms
5. Immune Support
6. Antioxidant Support
7. Bone Health
8. Heart Health
9. Liver Health
10. Metabolic Health
11. Ocular Health
12. Methylation Support
13. Lipotropic Factors
14. Inflammation Control
15. Glycation Control
16. Bioflavonoid Profile
17. Phenolic Compounds
18. Potential Toxicities

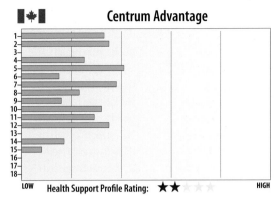

Centrum Advantage

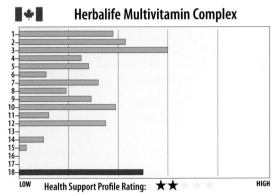

Herbalife Multivitamin Complex

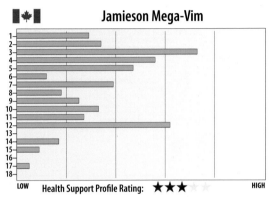

Jamieson Mega-Vim

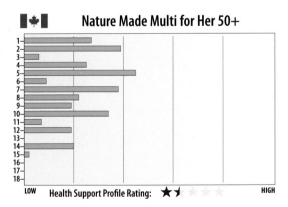

Nature Made Multi for Her 50+

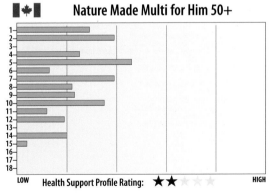

Nature Made Multi for Him 50+

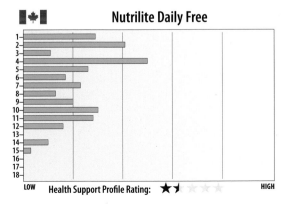

Nutrilite Daily Free

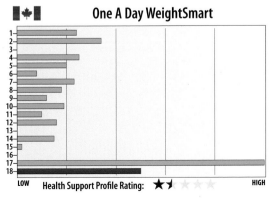

One A Day WeightSmart

Health Support Graph Legend

1. Completeness
2. Potency
3. Mineral Forms
4. Vitamin E Forms
5. Immune Support
6. Antioxidant Support
7. Bone Health
8. Heart Health
9. Liver Health
10. Metabolic Health
11. Ocular Health
12. Methylation Support
13. Lipotropic Factors
14. Inflammation Control
15. Glycation Control
16. Bioflavonoid Profile
17. Phenolic Compounds
18. Potential Toxicities

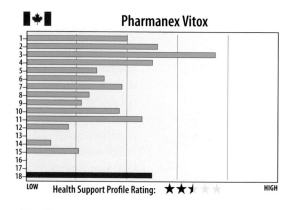

Pharmanex Vitox

Health Support Profile Rating: ★★⯪ ☆ ☆

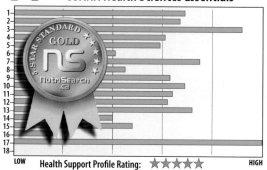

USANA Health Sciences Essentials

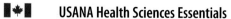

Health Support Profile Rating: ★★★★★

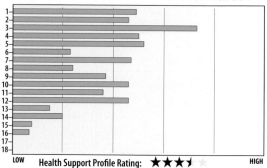

Webber Naturals MultiSure For Men 50+

Health Support Profile Rating: ★★★⯪ ☆

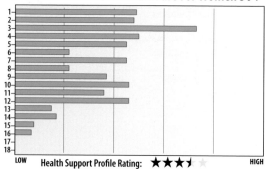

Webber Naturals MultiSure For Women 50+

Health Support Profile Rating: ★★★⯪ ☆

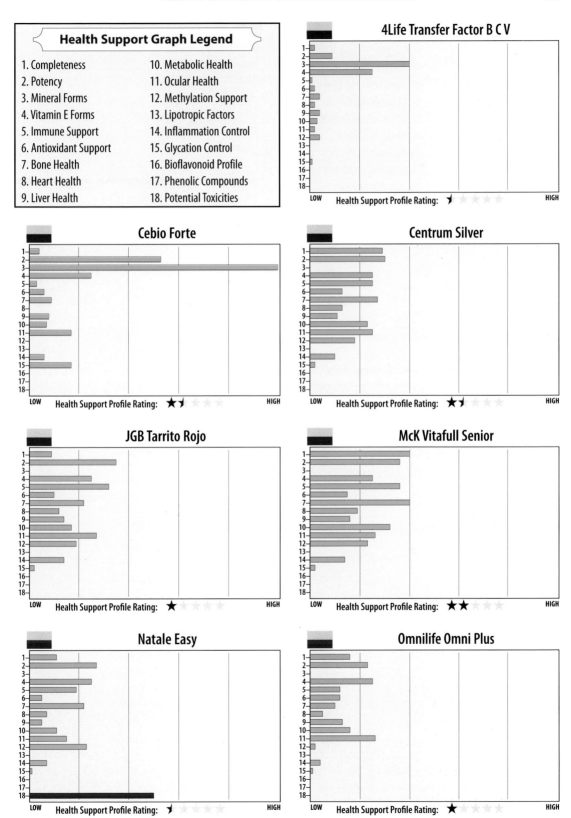

Health Support Graph Legend

1. Completeness
2. Potency
3. Mineral Forms
4. Vitamin E Forms
5. Immune Support
6. Antioxidant Support
7. Bone Health
8. Heart Health
9. Liver Health
10. Metabolic Health
11. Ocular Health
12. Methylation Support
13. Lipotropic Factors
14. Inflammation Control
15. Glycation Control
16. Bioflavonoid Profile
17. Phenolic Compounds
18. Potential Toxicities

4Life Transfer Factor B C V
LOW   Health Support Profile Rating: ⭐   HIGH

Cebio Forte
LOW   Health Support Profile Rating: ⭐⭐   HIGH

Centrum Silver
LOW   Health Support Profile Rating: ⭐⭐   HIGH

JGB Tarrito Rojo
LOW   Health Support Profile Rating: ⭐   HIGH

McK Vitafull Senior
LOW   Health Support Profile Rating: ⭐⭐   HIGH

Natale Easy
LOW   Health Support Profile Rating: ⭐   HIGH

Omnilife Omni Plus
LOW   Health Support Profile Rating: ⭐   HIGH

Health Support Graph Legend

1. Completeness
2. Potency
3. Mineral Forms
4. Vitamin E Forms
5. Immune Support
6. Antioxidant Support
7. Bone Health
8. Heart Health
9. Liver Health

10. Metabolic Health
11. Ocular Health
12. Methylation Support
13. Lipotropic Factors
14. Inflammation Control
15. Glycation Control
16. Bioflavonoid Profile
17. Phenolic Compounds
18. Potential Toxicities

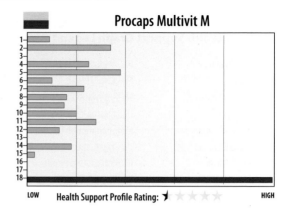

Procaps Multivit M

LOW   Health Support Profile Rating: ★ ★ ★ ★ ★   HIGH

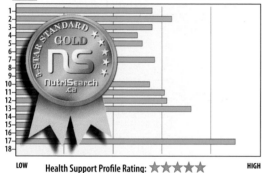

USANA Health Sciences Los Essentials*

LOW   Health Support Profile Rating: ★ ★ ★ ★ ★   HIGH

This product is not included in the Euromonitor International data, since it was not yet in the Colombian marketplace when the data was collected. We have included it, since it is a Five-Star, Gold Medal recipient.

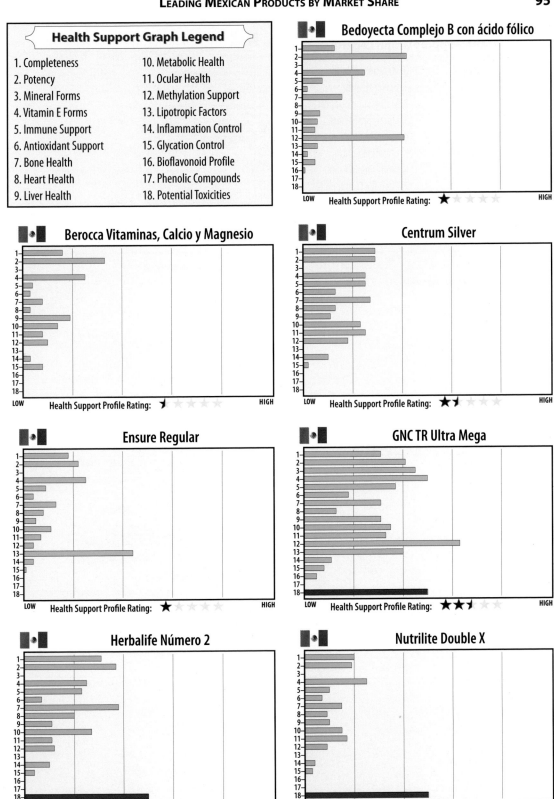

Health Support Graph Legend

1. Completeness
2. Potency
3. Mineral Forms
4. Vitamin E Forms
5. Immune Support
6. Antioxidant Support
7. Bone Health
8. Heart Health
9. Liver Health
10. Metabolic Health
11. Ocular Health
12. Methylation Support
13. Lipotropic Factors
14. Inflammation Control
15. Glycation Control
16. Bioflavonoid Profile
17. Phenolic Compounds
18. Potential Toxicities

Health Support Graph Legend

1. Completeness
2. Potency
3. Mineral Forms
4. Vitamin E Forms
5. Immune Support
6. Antioxidant Support
7. Bone Health
8. Heart Health
9. Liver Health
10. Metabolic Health
11. Ocular Health
12. Methylation Support
13. Lipotropic Factors
14. Inflammation Control
15. Glycation Control
16. Bioflavonoid Profile
17. Phenolic Compounds
18. Potential Toxicities

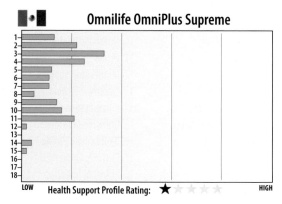

Omnilife OmniPlus Supreme

Health Support Profile Rating: ★☆☆☆☆   LOW ... HIGH

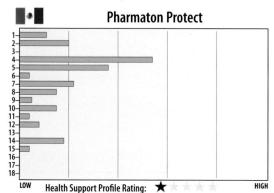

Pharmaton Protect

Health Support Profile Rating: ★☆☆☆☆   LOW ... HIGH

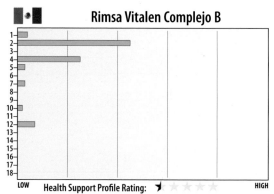

Rimsa Vitalen Complejo B

Health Support Profile Rating: ⯪☆☆☆☆   LOW ... HIGH

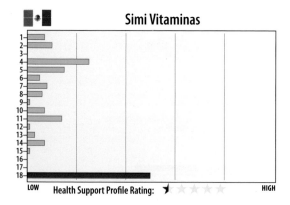

Simi Vitaminas

Health Support Profile Rating: ⯪☆☆☆☆   LOW ... HIGH

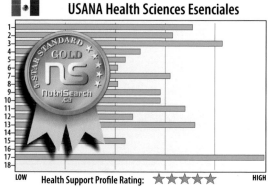

USANA Health Sciences Esenciales

Health Support Profile Rating: ★★★★★   LOW ... HIGH

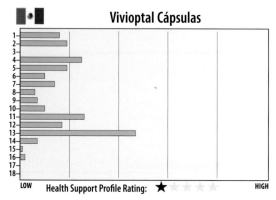

Vivioptal Cápsulas

Health Support Profile Rating: ★☆☆☆☆   LOW ... HIGH

Health Support Graph Legend

1. Completeness
2. Potency
3. Mineral Forms
4. Vitamin E Forms
5. Immune Support
6. Antioxidant Support
7. Bone Health
8. Heart Health
9. Liver Health
10. Metabolic Health
11. Ocular Health
12. Methylation Support
13. Lipotropic Factors
14. Inflammation Control
15. Glycation Control
16. Bioflavonoid Profile
17. Phenolic Compounds
18. Potential Toxicities

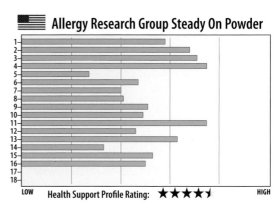

Allergy Research Group Steady On Powder

LOW   Health Support Profile Rating: ★★★★✦   HIGH

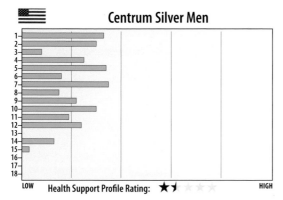

Centrum Silver Men

LOW   Health Support Profile Rating: ★✦ ☆ ☆ ☆   HIGH

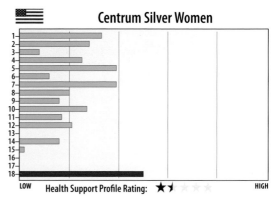

Centrum Silver Women

LOW   Health Support Profile Rating: ★✦ ☆ ☆ ☆   HIGH

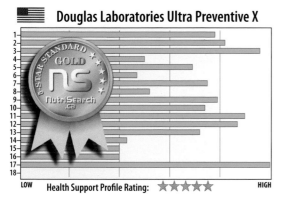

Douglas Laboratories Ultra Preventive X

LOW   Health Support Profile Rating: ★★★★★   HIGH

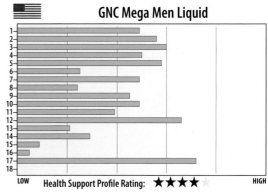

GNC Mega Men Liquid

LOW   Health Support Profile Rating: ★★★★ ☆   HIGH

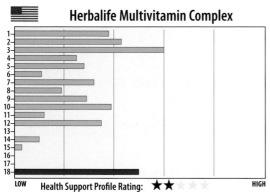

Herbalife Multivitamin Complex

LOW   Health Support Profile Rating: ★★ ☆ ☆ ☆   HIGH

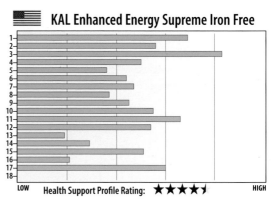

KAL Enhanced Energy Supreme Iron Free

LOW   Health Support Profile Rating: ★★★★✦   HIGH

Health Support Graph Legend

1. Completeness
2. Potency
3. Mineral Forms
4. Vitamin E Forms
5. Immune Support
6. Antioxidant Support
7. Bone Health
8. Heart Health
9. Liver Health
10. Metabolic Health
11. Ocular Health
12. Methylation Support
13. Lipotropic Factors
14. Inflammation Control
15. Glycation Control
16. Bioflavonoid Profile
17. Phenolic Compounds
18. Potential Toxicities

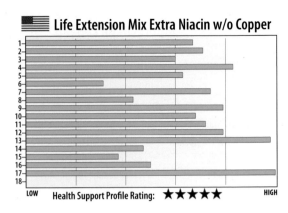

Life Extension Mix Extra Niacin w/o Copper

LOW   Health Support Profile Rating: ★★★★★   HIGH

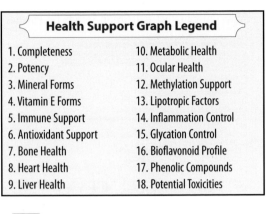

Melaleuca Vitality Men's

LOW   Health Support Profile Rating: ★★★☆   HIGH

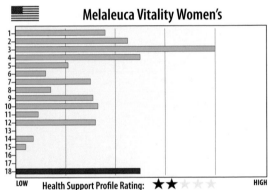

Melaleuca Vitality Women's

LOW   Health Support Profile Rating: ★★☆☆☆   HIGH

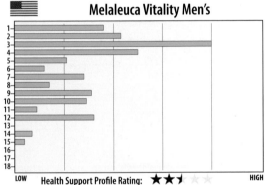

Natrol My Favorite Multiple Iron Free

LOW   Health Support Profile Rating: ★★★★☆   HIGH

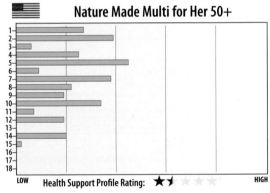

Nature Made Multi for Her 50+

LOW   Health Support Profile Rating: ★☆   HIGH

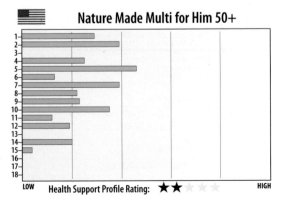

Nature Made Multi for Him 50+

LOW   Health Support Profile Rating: ★★☆☆☆   HIGH

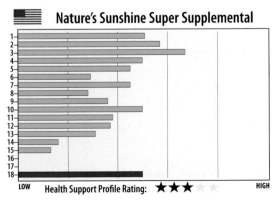

Nature's Sunshine Super Supplemental

LOW   Health Support Profile Rating: ★★★☆☆   HIGH

Health Support Graph Legend

1. Completeness
2. Potency
3. Mineral Forms
4. Vitamin E Forms
5. Immune Support
6. Antioxidant Support
7. Bone Health
8. Heart Health
9. Liver Health
10. Metabolic Health
11. Ocular Health
12. Methylation Support
13. Lipotropic Factors
14. Inflammation Control
15. Glycation Control
16. Bioflavonoid Profile
17. Phenolic Compounds
18. Potential Toxicities

Nutrilite Daily Free
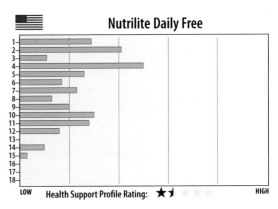
LOW   Health Support Profile Rating: ★★   HIGH

One A Day Men's 50+ Advantage
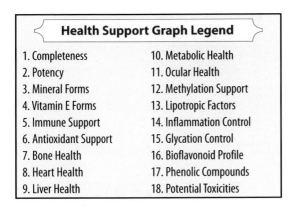
LOW   Health Support Profile Rating: ★★   HIGH

One A Day Women's 50+ Advantage
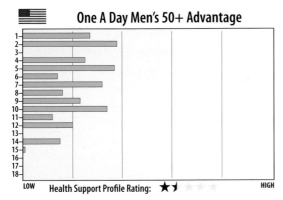
LOW   Health Support Profile Rating: ★★   HIGH

Pharmanex Vitox
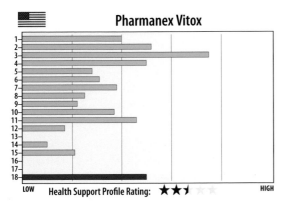
LOW   Health Support Profile Rating: ★★★   HIGH

Shaklee Vita-Lea Gold Vitamin K
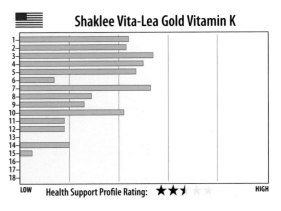
LOW   Health Support Profile Rating: ★★★   HIGH

Solgar Female Multiple
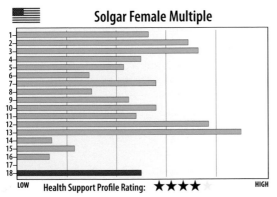
LOW   Health Support Profile Rating: ★★★★   HIGH

Solgar Male Multiple
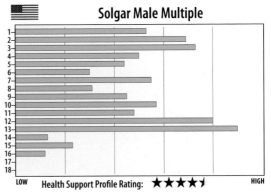
LOW   Health Support Profile Rating: ★★★★★   HIGH

1. Completeness	10. Metabolic Health
2. Potency	11. Ocular Health
3. Mineral Forms	12. Methylation Support
4. Vitamin E Forms	13. Lipotropic Factors
5. Immune Support	14. Inflammation Control
6. Antioxidant Support	15. Glycation Control
7. Bone Health	16. Bioflavonoid Profile
8. Heart Health	17. Phenolic Compounds
9. Liver Health	18. Potential Toxicities

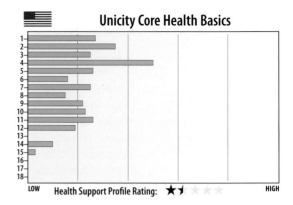

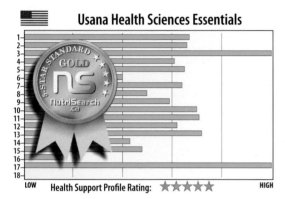

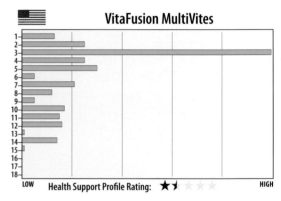

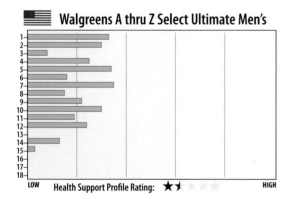

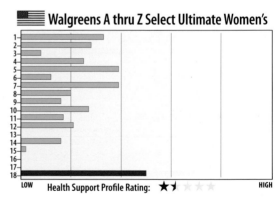

CHAPTER TEN:

PRODUCT RATINGS

Table 8: Canadian Products in Alphabetical Order

Manufacturer & Product Name	Rating
ADRIEN GAGNON MULTI ACTIVE MEN	★½
ADRIEN GAGNON MULTI ACTIVE MEN 50+	★★
ADRIEN GAGNON MULTI ACTIVE WOMEN	★½
ADRIEN GAGNON MULTI ACTIVE WOMEN 50+	★★
ADRIEN GAGNON MULTI ADULTS	★
ADVANCED NUTRITION BY ZAHLER (SEE ZAHLER)	
AGELOSS (SEE NATURE'S PLUS)	
ALBI NATURALS MULTI VITA-MINERAL	★★★
ALBI NATURALS SUPER ROCKY	★★½
AOR ADVANCED SERIES MULTI BASICS COMPLETE	★★★★½
AOR ADVANCED SERIES MULTI BASICS-3	★★★½
AOR CLASSIC SERIES ESSENTIAL MIX	★★★★
AWARENESS LIFE DAILY COMPLETE	★★½
BE TRUE (SEE TRUESTAR HEALTH)	
BIO-ACTIF PHYTOBEC	★½
BIOCLINIC NATURALS BIOFOUNDATION-G	★★★★½
BIOMÉDIC ADVANTAGE	★★
BIOMÉDIC FORMULE FORTE	★
BIOX ULTIMATE ONCE A DAY	★★★★
BODYBREAK ENERGY & VITALITY	★★
BODYBREAK SILVER 50+	★★
BODYBREAK TOTAL HEALTH	★★
CANPREV ADULT MULTI	★★★★
CANPREV IMMUNO MULTI	★★★★½
CENTRUM	½
CENTRUM ADVANTAGE	★★
CENTRUM FLAVOUR BURST CHEWS	★
CENTRUM FOR MEN	★
CENTRUM FOR WOMEN	★
CENTRUM FORTE	★
CENTRUM PERFORMANCE	★
CENTRUM SELECT 50+	★½
CENTRUM SELECT 50+ CHEWABLES	★
DEE CEE LABORATORIES (SEE DC)	
DOCTOR'S CHOICE (SEE ENZYMATIC THERAPY)	

Manufacturer & Product Name	Rating
DOUGLAS LABORATORIES ULTRA BALANCE III	★★★★½
DOUGLAS LABORATORIES ULTRA BALANCE III CAPSULES	★★★★
DOUGLAS LABORATORIES ULTRA BALANCE III WITH COPPER & IRON	★★★★½
DOUGLAS LABORATORIES ULTRA BALANCE III WITH IRON	★★★★½
DOUGLAS LABORATORIES ULTRA PREVENTIVE X VEGETARIAN CAPSULES	★★★★½
DR. BEN KIM NATURAL HEALTH SOLUTIONS COMPREHENSIVE FORMULA	★★
ENEREX SONA MULTI ATHLETES & 55 PLUS	★★★½
ENEREX SONA MULTI ORIGINAL	★★★
ENEREX SONA PURE	★★★
ENEREX SUPREME ONCE-A-DAY	★★★
ENEREX SUPREME TWICE-A-DAY	★★★
ENIVA VIBE APPLE	★★
ENIVA VIBE FRUIT SENSATION	★★
EQUATE CENTURY ADVANCE	★½
EQUATE CENTURY COMPLETE	½
EQUATE CENTURY PLUS	★
EQUATE CENTURY PREFERENCE	★
EQUATE CENTURY PREMIUM	★
EQUATE CENTURY SILVER	★½
EQUATE MEN'S 50+	★½
EQUATE WOMEN'S 50+	½
EQUATE WOMEN'S FORMULA	½
ESPECIALLY YOURS (SEE NATURE'S PLUS)	
EXACT ESSENTRA BALANCE	½
EXACT ESSENTRA ELITE	★
EXACT ESSENTRA FORTE	★
EXACT ESSENTRA PERFORMA	★
EXACT ESSENTRA PLATINUM	★
EXACT MULTI MAX 1	★★½
EXACT VITAL 1	½
EXACT VITAL 1 DAILY MEN'S 50+ FORMULA	★½
EXACT VITAL 1 MEN'S FORMULA	★½
GENESTRA ALMOND LIQUID VITE MIN	★★★
GENESTRA LIQUID MULTI VITE MIN	★★

Manufacturer & Product Name	Rating
Genestra Maxum Multi Vite	★★½
Genestra Multi Vite	★★
Genestra Super Orti Vite	★★
Genestra Vite Min Mix Vitamin Powder	★★★★
Genuine Health Multi+ Complete	★★★
Genuine Health Multi+ Daily Energy	★★½
Genuine Health Multi+ Daily Glow	★★★
Genuine Health Multi+ Daily Joy	★★★½
Genuine Health Multi+ Daily Trim	★★★
Herbalife Multivitamin Complex	★★
Highland Laboratories (see Mt. Angel Vitamin Company)	
Inno-Vite Formula H.H.	★★½
Jamieson Mega-Vim	★★★
Jamieson Power Vitamins for Men	★★½
Jamieson Vita Slim	★★
Jamieson Vita-Vim for Women	★½
Jamieson Vita-Vim Healthy Heart	★½
Jamieson Vita-Vim Regular	★★
Jamieson Vita-Vim Super	★★½
Jean-Marc Brunet (see Le Naturiste)	
Jeunesse (see Nutrigen)	
Kirkland Signature Formula Forte for Men	★
Kirkland Signature Formula Forte for Women	★
Kirkland Signature Formula Forte Senior	★½
Le Naturiste ABC Plus Senior	★
Le Naturiste Vitaminol Men's Multivitamin	★½
Le Naturiste Vitaminol Multivitamin for Adults 50+	★½
Life Adult Multivitamins for People Over 50	½
Life Daily-One for Men 50+	★½
Life Daily-One for Women	½
Life Spectrum Advanced	★★
Life Spectrum Forte	★
Life Spectrum Gold for Adults Over 50	★½
Life Spectrum with Lutein	½
London Drugs Multi Complete	½
London Drugs Multi Plus	★
London Drugs Multi Vitamin & Minerals	★
London Drugs One Tablet Daily Adults 50+	★½
Mauves (see Trophic)	
Multibionta Probiotic Multivitamin	½
Multibionta Probiotic Multivitamin 50+	½

Manufacturer & Product Name	Rating
MultiSure (see Webber Naturals)	
N.F. Formulas (see Integrative Therapeutics)	
Nāka Nutri Multi	★★★½
Nāka Nutri Multi for Men	★★★★
Nāka Nutri Multi for Women	★★★★
Natural Factors Hi Potency Multi	★★★½
Natural Factors MultiFactors Women's	★★★★½
Natural Factors MultiFactors Women's 50+	★★★★½
Nature Made Multi for Her 50+	★★½
Nature Made Multi for Him 50+	★★
Nature's Bounty ABC Plus Senior	★
Nature's Bounty Mega Vita-Min	★★★½
Nature's Harmony Adult Chewable Superior One-Per-Day	★★★½
Nature's Harmony High Potency One-Per-Day	★★★
Nature's Harmony Superior One-Per-Day	★★½
New Roots Multi	★★★★
New Roots Multi-Max	★★★★
New Roots Multi-MaxImmune	★★★★½
Nu-Life The Ultimate One Men 50+	★★★★½
Nu-Life The Ultimate One Women 50+	★★★★½
Nutra Therapeutics (see Adëeva)	
Nutribetics Multi-Vitamin	★★★
Nutrilite Daily Free	★★½
Nutrition House Men's Multi Extra	★★★★½
Nutrition House Multi-Vitamin Extra	★★★½
Nutrition House Women's Multi Extra	★★★★½
One A Day for Men	★★½
One A Day for Men 50 Plus	★★½
One A Day for Women	½
One A Day for Women 50 Plus	½
One A Day WeightSmart	★★½
Optima Multivit & Mineralex	★★
Option+ Multi	★
Option+ Multi Adult	★★½
Option+ Multi Forte	★
Option+ Multi Forte Senior	★
Organika Multiple Vitamins with Minerals	★
Organika One Daily	★★
Personnelle Complete	½
Personnelle Forte	★
Personnelle Senior	★

Manufacturer & Product Name	Rating
Personnelle Superia	★
Pharmacists Selection Multivitamin Multimineral	½
Pharmacists Selection Multivitamin Multimineral Plus	★
Pharmanex Vitox	★★½
Pharmax Adult Formula	★★★
Phytobec	★½
Prairie Naturals Multi-Force	★★★★
Prairie Naturals Multi-Force Iron Free	★★★★½
Prairie Naturals MultiForce ORAC	★★½
Progressive Active Men	★★★★
Progressive Active Women	★★★★
Progressive Adult Men	★★★½
Progressive Adult Women	★★★½
Progressive Men 50+	★★★★
Progressive Women's 50+	★★★★
Purity Products Perfect Multi Super Greens for Canada	★★★★½
Purpose (See Creating Wellness)	
Quest Adult Chewables	★½
Quest Mature Men 50+ His Daily One	★★½
Quest Mature Women 50+ Her Daily One	★★½
Quest Maximum Once A Day	★★★½
Quest Men His Daily One	★★★½
Quest Premium Multi-Cap	★½
Quest Premium Multi-Cap iron-free	★★
Quest Super Once A Day	★★½
Quest Women Her Daily One	★★
Quest Women Her Daily One Chewable	★½
Réservé 50+ Senior Formula	★
Réservé Forte Formula	★
Réservé Regular Formula	½
Rexall (see Sundown Naturals)	
Rexall Adult Formula	½
Rexall Adults 50+ Formula	★½
Rexall Complete	½
Rexall Complete for Adults 50+	★
Rexall Complete Forte	★
Rexall Complete Premium	★
Rexall Multivitamin + Multimineral Forte	★
Rexall Women's Formula	½
Sangster's Choice Apex	★

Manufacturer & Product Name	Rating
Sangster's Men's Choice	★★★½
Sangster's Women's Choice	★★★
Selekta Multi's (w/o Copper & Iron)	★★★
Shaklee Vita-Lea Gold with Vitamin K	★★★½
Shaklee Vita-Lea Gold without Vitamin K	★★★½
Shaklee Vita-Lea Iron Formula	★★
Shaklee Vita-Lea Without Iron Formula	★★
S īsū Multi Vi Min	★★
S īsū Optimal Health Multi 1	★★★
S īsū Supreme Multivitamin	★★★½
S īsū Supreme Multivitamin 50+	★★★★
S īsū Supreme Multivitamin with Iron	★★★
SomaLife SomaVit Plus	★★★
Swiss Adult Chewable Multi Vitamin & Mineral	★★
Swiss Adult Multi One Formula	★★
Swiss Iron Free Vege	★★★½
Swiss One	★
Swiss One 25	★½
Swiss One 50	★★½
Swiss One 80	★★★
Swiss Total One Antioxidant	★★½
Swiss Total One Men	★★½
Swiss Total One Men 50+	★★½
Swiss Total One Sport	★★½
Swiss Total One Women	★★
Swiss Total One Women 50+	★★½
Tanta Formula Forte Senior	★
The Results Company (see Vitamost)	
The Synergy Company (see Pure Synergy)	
Trophic Complete One	★★½
Trophic Men's 50+	★★★★½
Trophic Men's Ultra Complete	★★★★½
Trophic Vita Balance & Minero Balance	★★½
Trophic Women's 50+	★★★★½
Trophic Women's Ultra Complete	★★★★½
Truehope EMPowerplus	★★★
Truestar Health TrueBASICS Solo	★★★★★
Usana Health Sciences Essentials — *Editor's Choice Award*	★★★★★
Vita-Complete AA	★½
Vita-Complete Vita29	★
Vitalux Healthy Eyes	★★

MANUFACTURER & PRODUCT NAME	RATING
VITALUX TIMED RELEASE MULTIVITAMIN/ MULTIMINERAL	★★
VITAMIN CODE (SEE GARDEN OF LIFE)	
VITAMINOL (SEE LE NATURISTE)	
VITAZAN PROFESSIONAL MULTI	★★★
VIVITAS WOMAN ONE FOR HER	★★
VIVITAS WOMAN ONE FOR HER 50+	★★½
WAMPOLE ADULT MULTIVITAMIN CHEWABLE	½
WEBBER NATURALS MULTI VITAMIN	★
WEBBER NATURALS MULTISURE FOR MEN	★★★½
WEBBER NATURALS MULTISURE FOR MEN 50+	★★★½
WEBBER NATURALS MULTISURE FOR WOMEN	★★★
WEBBER NATURALS MULTISURE FOR WOMEN 50+	★★★½
WEBBER NATURALS MULTISURE HEALTHY AGING	★★★
WESTCOAST NATURALS MULTI-ONE	★★½

Table 9: Colombian Products in Alphabetical Order

Manufacturer & Product Name	Rating
4Life Transfer Factor B C V	½
Amway (see Nutrilite)	
Bionutricol Numax	★★½
BPM EstresSIN	½
Brainy (see Robinson Pharma)	
Caliproy (see Natural Care Pharmaceutics)	
Cebio Forte	★½
Centrum	★
Centrum Silver	★½
Colmed International Polivitaminas y Minerales	½
Ensure Advance	½
Ensure Con Prebiotics FOS & Inulina	½
Enterex	½
Everyday Health Wellness Man	½
Everyday Health Wellness Woman	½
Finlay Vitacerebrina Next	½
Frexen Capsules	½
Frexen Capsules Plus	½
Funat Funasure	½
Funat Transfermune Forte	½
Funat Vitasource	½
Genomma Lab ShotB	½
GNC Mega Men	★★½
GNC Mega Teen	★
GNC Ultra Mega Women's	★★½
Good'n Natural Multi Vitamin Formula	★
Good'n Natural Ultra Man	★½
Good'n Natural Ultra Woman	★★½
Herbalife Fórmula 1 Batido Nutricional	½
Herbalife Fórmula 2 Complejo Multivitamínico	½
JGB Tarrito Rojo	★
La Santé Vital 2B Healthy Multivitaminico	★½
La Santé Vital Nutri Men	½
Laboratorios Best Coboral Z	½
Ledmar Neurolife	★
Mason Natural VitaTrum	★
McK Kola Granulada	★½
McK Vitafull	★½
McK Vitafull Senior	★★

Manufacturer & Product Name	Rating
Natale Easy	½
Natural Care Pharmaceutics Calciproy	★½
Natural Medicine Multivitamin	½
Naturcol Malta Shake MX	★
Nature's Sunshine Mega-Chel	★
Nature's Sunshine Solstic	½
Neurolife (see Ledmar)	
Numax (see Bionutricol)	
Nutrabiotics Metabessens	★★★
Nutrabiotics Multiessens Vitaminas & Minerales	★★★★★
Nutrilite Daily	½
Nutrilite Double X	★★★½
Omnilife OmniPlus	★
Orthomol Immun	★★
Orthomol Sport	★★½
Orthomol Vital F	★★
Orthomol Vital M	★★
Pharmanex LifePak	★★★
Pharmaton Vitality	½
Procaps Multivit M	½
Robinson Pharma Brainy	★
Sabor Natural Milivit	½
ShotB (see Genomma Lab)	
Solaray Spectro	★★★½
Sundown Naturals Adult Multivitamin Gummies	★½
Sundown Naturals Advanced Formula Sun Vite	★
Sustagen Nutrición + Completa	½
UPN Megaplex	½
USANA Health Sciences Los Essentials *Editor's Choice Award*	★★★★★
Vitalor Con Omega 3	★½
Z-BEC Advance	★

Table 10: Méxican Products in Alphabetical Order

Manufacturer & Product Name	Rating
AFG Plus	½
Alpha Betic	★★½
Amway (see Nutrilite)	
Anavit	★
Bedoyecta Complejo B con ácido fólico	★
Berocca Vitaminas, Calcio y Magnesio	½
Biokonic Vitaminas y Minerales	½
Biometrix A-OX	★
Biometrix Cápsulas	½
Biomiral Prodia-Vit	★
Bioprotect Vitaminas y Minerales	½
Bioretin	★★½
Centrum Performance	★
Centrum Silver	★★½
Centrum Vitaminas y Minerales	★
CMD Productos Naturales Diabenel	★
CMD Productos Naturales Diabenel Max	★
CMD Productos Naturales Vitamix	½
Cure Pharma VitaVid	½
Cure Pharma VitaVid Silver	½
Cyntelle 03	½
Diabion	★
Dr. Mann Pharma Vivioptal	★
Elevit	★
Energy Pack	½
Ensure Advance	½
Ensure Plus	★
Ensure Regular	★
Equate Power Plus	★
Farmacom Vitaminas, Minerales, Ginkgo Biloba y Panax Ginseng	★
Fasa Vitaminas Para Abuelitos	★
Fasa Vitaminas Para Adultos	½
Fasa Vitaminas, Minerales, Power Plus	★
Fortalite	½
Gelcavit Geriátrico	½
Gelcavit Mulier	★
Gelcavit Multivitamínico con Minerales	½
Gelcavit Q-10	½

Manufacturer & Product Name	Rating
Gelcavit Vitaminas, Minerales, Panax Ginseng y Gingko Biloba	½
Geramin Caps B12	½
GNC Mega Men	★★½
GNC Mega Men 50 Plus	★★
GNC Mega Men Sport	★★
GNC Platinum Years	★★½
GNC TR Ultra Mega	★★★½
GNC Ultra Mega Gold	★★★½
GNC Women's	★★½
GNC Women's Ultra Mega	★★
GNC Women's Ultra Mega 50 Plus	★★½
Herbalife Número 2	★
Kirkland Signature Vitaminas, Minerales y Luteina	★
Kirkland Signature Vitaminas, Minerales, Ginkgo Biloba y Panax Ginseng	★
Maxivit	½
Medisource Multivitamínico Multimineral	★
Medsulab Multivitamínico para +55	★
Medsulab Multivitamínico para Hombres	½
Medsulab Multivitamínico para Mujeres	½
Megavital Q-10	½
Member's Mark Vitaminas, Minerales	★
Menoflavin	½
Multibionta Probioticos, Vitaminas y Minerales	½
Nanavit	½
Naturex MaxiB GS	½
Naturex Vitrex G	½
Nutragold One-a-Day Essential	★
Nutragold Ultra Man	★
Nutragold V & M Ultra	★
Nutricion 2000 Vital-Mi	★
Nutrilite (Amway) Daily	½
Nutrilite (Amway) Double X	½
Omnilife OmniPlus Supreme	★
Optimum Nutrition Opti-Men	★★★½
Optimum Nutrition Opti-Women	★★★½
Pharmaton Cápsulas	½
Pharmaton Protect	★
Piñalim GN + Vida	½
Polibetic Vitaminas y Minerales	★

Manufacturer & Product Name	Rating
Power Plus Tabletas	★
ReGenesis Vitaminas, Minerales con Ácido Fólico y Omega 3	½
Retrovirón Energético	½
Revitrón Vitaminas y Minerales	½
Rimsa Vitalen Complejo B	½
Roca Vit Platinum	½
Roca Vit Platinum Pack IIII	½
Roca Vit Plus Q10	½
ShotB GS	½
Simi Vitaminas	½
Stresstabs 600 con Zinc	★
Sukrol Hombre	½
Sukrol Mujer	½
USANA Health Sciences Esenciales _Editor's Choice Award_	★★★★★
Vigorol Maxi Men	★
Vita Forte	★
Vital Fuerte	½
Vital Fuerte H3	½
Viterra Plus	½
Vivioptal Cápsulas	★

Table 11: US Products in Alphabetical Order

Manufacturer & Product Name	Rating
1st Endurance Multi-V	★★★
1st Step for Energy 71 Vitamins and Minerals	★½
21st Century Mega Multi for Men	★★½
21st Century Mega Multi for Women	★★★
21st Century One Daily Adults 50+	★½
21st Century One Daily Cholesterol Health	★
21st Century One Daily Maximum	½
21st Century One Daily Men's 50+	★½
21st Century One Daily Men's Health	★
21st Century One Daily Women's	½
21st Century One Daily Women's 50+	★½
21st Century Sentry	★
21st Century Sentry Cardio Support	★
21st Century Sentry Perform	★
21st Century Sentry Senior	★
4Life Multiplex	★★½
Absolute Nutrition Uno Diario Hombres	★
Absolute Nutrition Uno Diario Mujeres	½
Action Labs Action-Tabs Made For Men	★½
Adëeva All-In-One	★★★½
Advanced Nutrition By Zahler (see Zahler)	
Advanced Nutritional Innovations (ANI) CoralAdvantage	★★
Advanced Nutritional Innovations (ANI) Joint Health	★★★★
Advocare CorePlex Chewable	★½
Advocare CorePlex with Iron	★★★½
Advocare V100 Multivitamin	★½
Agel Min	★★
Ageloss (see Nature's Plus)	
All One Active Seniors	★★★★½
All One Fruit Antioxidant	★★★★
All One Green Phyto Base	★★★★
All One Original Formula	★★★★
All One Rice Base	★★★★½
All One Tablets for Travel	★★★½
Allergy Research Group Multi-Vi-Min	★★
Allergy Research Group Multi-Vi-Min without Copper & Iron	★★
Allergy Research Group Steady On Powder	★★★★½
alpha betic Multivitamin Plus Extended Energy	★★★
AlternaVites Multivitamins & Minerals	★★½
American Health Nutri-Mega	★★★
American Nutrition Active Man's Formula	★★★★
American Nutrition Active Woman's Multi	★★★★½
American Nutrition Life Essentials	★★★★½
Anabolic Laboratories Aved-Eze Multi	★★
Anabolic Laboratories Aved-Multi	★★½
Anabolic Laboratories Aved-Multi Iron Free	★★½
Anabolic Laboratories Multigel Caps	★★★½
Analytical Research Labs Endo-Mins	★½
Analytical Research Labs Megapan	★½
Apex 50 Plus Multivitamin	★★½
Apex Performance Multivitamin	★★★½
Apex Women's Multivitamin	★★
Applied Nutriceuticals Complete-Balance	★½
Ariix Vitamins & Minerals	★★★★★½
AST Sports Science Multi Pro 32X	★★★★½
Balance Nutraceuticals MultiBalance No Iron	★★★★★½
Balance Nutraceuticals MultiBalance Plus Iron	★★★★★
Be True (see Truestar Health)	
Be Well Complete Multivitamin	★★★★★½
Beachbody Nutritionals ActiVit	★★★
Beachbody Shakeology (Chocolate)	½
Beachbody Shakeology (Vanilla, Greenberry)	★
Beyond Health Multi-Vitamin Formula	★★★★★½
BioGenesis MultiGreens	★★★★★½
BioGenesis Premiere Greens Multi	★
BioGenesis Ultra Genesis	★★★★
BioGenesis Ultra Genesis without Iron	★★★★
BioGenesis Ultra Genesis without Iron & Copper	★★★★
Bio-Life Naturals Super Bio-Balance	★★★½
Bio-Lumin Essense Daily Essense	★★★½
Bio-Lumin Essense Living Essense	★
Biotics Research Bio Multi-Plus	★★½
Biotics Research Bio Multi-Plus Iron and Copper Free	★★
Biotics Research Bio Multi-Plus Iron Free	★★
Biotics Research Bio-Trophic Plus	★
Biotics Research Equi-Fem	★★★

Manufacturer & Product Name	Rating
Biotics Research Equi-Fem Iron and Copper Free	★★★½
Biotics Research ProMulti-Plus	★★★★½
Blueberry Health Sciences Essentials Premium	☆☆☆☆☆
Bluebonnet Age-less Choice for Men 50+	★★★★½
Bluebonnet Age-less Choice for Women 50+	★★★★½
Bluebonnet Ladies' Choice Caplets	★★★★½
Bluebonnet Maxi One Caplets	★★★½
Bluebonnet Maxi Two Caplets	★★★★
Bluebonnet Men's Choice Caplets	★★★★½
Bluebonnet Multi One Vcaps	★★½
Bluebonnet Multi-Vita Softgels	★★★
Bluebonnet Super Earth Multinutrient Formula	★★★★
Bluebonnet Super Vita-CoQ10 Formula Caplets	★★★★½
Bluebonnet Veggie Choice Caplets	★★★★½
Body Rewards Daily Multi	★★★
Body Wise Right Choice AM/PM	★★★★½
Botanic Choice Mega Multi Vitamin	★★★
Botanic Choice Whole Foods Power Multi	★★½
Bronson Advanced Mature Gold	★★½
Bronson All Insurance Vitamin Powder	★★★★
Bronson Chewable Vitamin & Mineral	★★
Bronson Daily Multi + Joint Support	★½
Bronson Fortified Vitamin & Mineral Insurance Formula	★★
Bronson GTC Formula	★★
Bronson GTC Formula #2	★
Bronson Mature Formula	★½
Bronson Mature Formula Without Iron	★★
Bronson Mega Multi Softcaps	★★
Bronson Men's Complete Formula	★★★
Bronson Omega Complete for Men	★★★★
Bronson Omega Complete For Women	★★★★
Bronson Performance Edge for Men	★★★
Bronson Performance Edge for Women	★★★
Bronson The Bronson Formula	★★
Bronson The Woman's Formula	★½
Bronson Therapeutic Formula	★
Bronson Vegi Source	★★★★½
Bronson Vitamin & Mineral Formula	★½

Manufacturer & Product Name	Rating
Bronson Vitamin & Mineral Insurance Formula	★★★
BSC Multi-VMA	★★★
Buried Treasure Active 55 Plus	★★★★
Buried Treasure Daily Nutrition	★★★
Buried Treasure VM-100 Complete	★★★★★½
Burns Drugs Multi-Max with Lutein	★★
Carlson ACES Gold	★★½
Carlson Fish Oil Multi	★★½
Carlson Mini-Multi	★½
Carlson Super 1 Daily	★★★
Carlson Super 2 Daily	★★★★½
Centrum Adults	★
Centrum Flavor Burst Chew	★
Centrum Flavor Burst Drink Mix	★½
Centrum Silver Adults 50+	★
Centrum Silver Men	★½
Centrum Silver Women	★½
Centrum Women	★
Century Systems Miracle 2000	★★★★
Cooper Complete Basic One Iron Free	★★½
Cooper Complete Basic One With Iron	★★★★½
Cooper Complete Elite Athlete	★★★★
Cooper Complete Iron Free	★★★★
Cooper Complete With Iron	★★★★½
Country Life Beyond Food	★★★★½
Country Life Chewable Adult Multi	★★
Country Life Daily Multi-Sorb	★★★½
Country Life Daily Total One	★★★½
Country Life Essential Life	★★★½
Country Life Liquid Multi	★★★★
Country Life Max for Men	★★★★
Country Life Max for Men Vegetarian Caps	★★★★
Country Life Maxine Iron-Free	★★★★
Country Life Maxi-Sorb Superior Multiple	★★★★½
Country Life Multi-100	★★★
Country Life Multi-Sorb Maxine	★★★★½
Country Life Multi-Sorb Maxine Vegetarian Capsules	★★★★½
Country Life Realfood Organics Men's Daily Nutrition	★
Country Life Realfood Organics Ultimate Daily Nutrition	★½

Manufacturer & Product Name	Rating
Country Life Realfood Organics Women's Daily Nutrition	★
Country Life Realfood Organics Your Daily Nutrition	★
Country Life Seniority Multivitamin	★★½
Country Life Vegetarian Support	★★★
Creating Wellness Purpose Vitalizing Men's Multi	★
Creating Wellness Purpose Vitalizing Women's Multi	★
CTD Labs Multi-elite	★★★★
CVS Pharmacy Daily Multiple	½
CVS Pharmacy Daily Multiple for Men	★½
CVS Pharmacy Daily Multiple for Women	★
CVS Pharmacy Daily Multiple Plus Minerals	½
CVS Pharmacy Spectravite	★
CVS Pharmacy Spectravite Senior	★
Cyto-Charge Life Assurance	★★★
D'Adamo Personalized Nutrition Exakta	★
DaVinci Laboratories of Vermont Daily Best	★★★
DaVinci Laboratories of Vermont Daily Best Ultra	★★★½
DaVinci Laboratories of Vermont Omni	★★
DaVinci Laboratories of Vermont Spectra	★★★★½
DaVinci Laboratories of Vermont Spectra Infinite Nutrition	★★★★★
DaVinci Laboratories of Vermont Spectra Man	★★★★½
DaVinci Laboratories of Vermont Spectra Multi Age	★★★★
DaVinci Laboratories of Vermont Spectra Senior	★★★★½
DaVinci Laboratories of Vermont Spectra Without Copper & Iron	★★★★
DaVinci Laboratories of Vermont Spectra Woman	★★★★
DaVinci Laboratories of Vermont Ultimate Spectra	★★★★★
DC Formula 19	★★½
DC Formula 249	★★½
DC Formula 360	★
DC Formula 75	★★½
DC Formula 784	★

Manufacturer & Product Name	Rating
DC Formula 814	★½
DC Vita-Men	★★★
DC Vita-Women	★★½
Dee Cee Laboratories (see DC)	
Designs for Health Complete Multi	★★★★½
Designs for Health Complete Multi with Copper and Iron	★★★★½
Designs for Health Metabolic Synergy	★★★★½
Designs for Health Twice Daily Multi	★★★★
Designs for Health Vitavescence (Packets)	★★★★
Doctor David Williams Daily Basics Plus	★★★★½
Doctor's Choice (see Enzymatic Therapy)	
Doctor's Nutrition Athletic Nutrients	★★★★½
Doctor's Nutrition Mega Vites Man	★★★★
Doctor's Nutrition Mega Vites Senior	★★★½
Doctor's Nutrition Mega Vites Without Copper & Iron	★★★★
Doctor's Nutrition Mega Vites Woman	★★★½
Don Lemmon's Multi-Nutrient Support Formula	★★★★
dōTerra Microplex VMz	★★
dotFit ActiveMV	★★★
Douglas Laboratories Added Protection III Without Copper	★★★★
Douglas Laboratories Added Protection III Without Copper & Iron	★★★★½
Douglas Laboratories Added Protection III Without Iron	★★★★½
Douglas Laboratories Basic Preventive 1	★★★★½
Douglas Laboratories Basic Preventive 2	★★★★½
Douglas Laboratories Basic Preventive 3	★★★★½
Douglas Laboratories Basic Preventive 4	★★★★½
Douglas Laboratories Basic Preventive 5	★★★★½
Douglas Laboratories Essential Basics	★★★★
Douglas Laboratories Multivite	★
Douglas Laboratories Ultra Fem	★★★★
Douglas Laboratories Ultra Genic	★★★½
Douglas Laboratories Ultra Preventive	★★★★★
Douglas Laboratories Ultra Preventive 2-A-Day	★★★★½
Douglas Laboratories Ultra Preventive Beta	★★★★½
Douglas Laboratories Ultra Preventive Beta with Copper	★★★★½

Manufacturer & Product Name	Rating
Douglas Laboratories Ultra Preventive Beta with Copper & Iron	★★★★½
Douglas Laboratories Ultra Preventive Forte-Chel	★★★★½
Douglas Laboratories Ultra Preventive III	★★★★½
Douglas Laboratories Ultra Preventive III Capsules	★★★½
Douglas Laboratories Ultra Preventive III Capsules with Copper	★★★★
Douglas Laboratories Ultra Preventive III with Copper	★★★★½
Douglas Laboratories Ultra Preventive III with Copper & Iron	★★★★½
Douglas Laboratories Ultra Preventive III with Iron	★★★★½
Douglas Laboratories Ultra Preventive III with Zinc Picolinate	★★★★½
Douglas Laboratories Ultra Preventive IX with Vitamin K	☆☆☆☆☆
Douglas Laboratories Ultra Preventive X	☆☆☆☆☆
Douglas Laboratories Ultra Vite 75 II	★★★
Douglas Laboratories Vitaworx	★★★★★
Dr. Cranton's PrimeNutrients	★★★★½
Dr. Donsbach Agua Vitae Mens	★★★★½
Dr. Donsbach Agua Vitae Unisex	★★★★½
Dr. Donsbach Agua Vitae Women's Formula	★★★★½
Dr. Fuhrman Gentle Care Formula	★★
Dr. Fuhrman Men's Daily Formula +D3	★★
Dr. Fuhrman Women's Daily Formula + D3	★★
Dr. Mercola Whole Food Multivitamin Plus Vital Minerals	★★★★★½
Dr. Rath's Vitacor Plus	★★
Dr. Sinatra Multivitamin for Men	★★★★½
Dr. Sinatra Multivitamin for Women	★★★★½
Dr. Weil Multivitamin & Antioxidant	★★★★½
Dr. Whitaker Forward	★★★★★½
Drinkables Liquid Multi Vitamins	★½
Drucker Labs IntraMax	★★★★½
Dymatize Nutrition Super Multi	★★★½
Eclectic Institute Optimum II, IV, VI Without Iron	★★★★
Eclectic Institute Vital Force	★★★★½
Eclectic Institute Vital Force Ultra-Caps	★★★★½
Eclectic Institute Vital Force without Iron	★★★★
ecoNugenics Men's Longevity Essentials Plus	★★★★½
ecoNugenics Women's Longevity Rhythms	★★★★½
Edom Labs Active Man's Formula	★★★★
Edom Labs Active Woman's Multi	★★★★½
Edom Labs Family-Vites	½
Edom Labs Natural Organic Formula 75	★★★
Edom Labs Natural Supervites	★★
Edom Labs Timed Release Ultra-Vites	★★★
Emergen-C Multi-Vitamin Plus	★½
Endurance Products Company Endur-VM	★
Endurance Products Company Endur-VM without Iron	★½
Energetix BioNutrient Complex	★★★★½
Enzymatic Therapy Doctor's Choice 45+ Women	★★★★★½
Enzymatic Therapy Doctor's Choice 50+ Men	★★★★½
Enzymatic Therapy Doctor's Choice Men	★★★★★½
Enzymatic Therapy Doctor's Choice Women	★★★★★½
Enzyme Labs Multi-Life	★★★½
Equate Active Adults 50+	★
Equate Adults Under 50	★
Equate Complete Multivitamin	½
Equate One Daily Men's Health	★★½
Equate One Daily Women's Health	★
Equate Women 50+	★★½
Equate Women's Pro-Active	★
Especially Yours (see Nature's Plus)	
Esteem Senior Total Man	★★★½
Esteem Senior Total Woman	★★★½
Esteem Total Man	★★★½
Esteem Total Woman	★★
Factor Nutrition Labs FOCUSfactor	★★
First Organics Daily Multiple	★★½
Flora Multi Caps	★★★
Food Research Vitamin & Mineral	★★½
Food Science of Vermont Daily Best	★★★
Food Science of Vermont Men's Superior	★★★★★½
Food Science of Vermont Senior's Superior	★★★★
Food Science of Vermont Superior Care	★★★★★½
Food Science of Vermont Superior Care Without Copper and Iron	★★★★
Food Science of Vermont Total Care	★★

Manufacturer & Product Name	Rating
Food Science of Vermont Ultimate Care	★★★★★
Food Science of Vermont Women's Superior	★★★★
Freeda Freedavite	★
Freeda Geri-Freeda	★★
Freeda Hi Kovite	★
Freeda Monocaps	★
Freeda Quintabs-M	★½
Freeda Quintabs-M Iron Free	★★
Freeda T-Vites	★½
Freeda Ultra Freeda	★★★
Freeda Ultra Freeda A Free	★★★
Freeda Ultra Freeda Iron Free	★★★½
Futurebiotics Hi Energy Multi for Men	★★★½
Futurebiotics Multi Vitamin Energy Plus for Women	★★
Futurebiotics Vegetarian Super Multi	★★★
Futurebiotics Vitomega Men	★★★½
Futurebiotics Vitomega Women	★★★½
Garden of Life Living Multi Optimal Formula	★★
Garden of Life Living Multi Optimal Men's Formula	★★½
Garden of Life Living Multi Optimal Women's Formula	★★
Garden of Life Vitamin Code 50 & Wiser Men	★★½
Garden of Life Vitamin Code 50 & Wiser Women	★★½
Garden of Life Vitamin Code Family	★★½
Garden of Life Vitamin Code Liquid Multivitamin Formula	★★★
Garden of Life Vitamin Code Men	★★
Garden of Life Vitamin Code Perfect Weight	★★½
Garden of Life Vitamin Code Raw One for Women	★½
Garden of Life Vitamin Code Raw One Men	★½
Garden of Life Vitamin Code Women	★★
Gary Null Super AM & Super PM Formulas	★★★★½
Gary Null Supreme Health	★★★★½
Genesis Super 100 Formula	★★★½
Genesis Today GenEssentials Organic Total Nutrition	★★
Geneva Levity+Plus	★★★
Geritol Complete	½
GNC be-WHOLE	★★★½

Manufacturer & Product Name	Rating
GNC Mega Men	★★★★
GNC Mega Men 50 Plus	★★★
GNC Mega Men 50+ One Daily	★★½
GNC Mega Men Energy & Metabolism	★★★★
GNC Mega Men Liquid	★★★★
GNC Mega Men Maximum Nutrition	★★★½
GNC Mega Men One Daily	★★½
GNC Mega Men Sport	★★★
GNC Solotron Chewable	★
GNC Ultra Mega Gold	★★★½
GNC Ultra Mega Green Men's	★★★½
GNC Ultra Mega Green Men's 50+	★★★½
GNC Ultra Mega Green Men's Sport	★★★½
GNC Ultra Mega Green Women's	★★★
GNC Ultra Mega Green Women's 50 Plus	★★★½
GNC Ultra Mega Green Women's Active	★★★
GNC Women's Ultra Mega	★★★
GNC Women's Ultra Mega 50 Plus	★★★
GNC Women's Ultra Mega 50 Plus One Daily	★★
GNC Women's Ultra Mega Active	★★★
GNC Women's Ultra Mega Bone Density Without Iron And Iodine	★★★½
GNC Women's Ultra Mega Energy & Metabolism	★★★½
GNC Women's Ultra Mega Maximum Nutrition	★★★
GNC Women's Ultra Mega One Daily	★★
GNC Women's Ultra Mega Without Iron and Iodine	★★★
GNLD Formula IV	★½
GNLD Vegetarian Multi	★★
Great American Products Green Supreme Multi	★★★½
Great American Products Liquid Master Multi	★½
Great American Products Master Green Multi	★★★★
Greens Today Men's Formula	★★★
Greens Today Original Formula	★★½
Greens Today Powerhouse Formula	★★½
Greens Today Vegan Formula	★★★
Health Direct Nature's Optimal Nutrition	★★★
Health First Multi-First	★★★½
H-E-B Complete	★
H-E-B One Daily for Men	★½

Manufacturer & Product Name	Rating
H-E-B One Daily for Women	★
H-E-B Ultimate Men's	★
H-E-B Ultimate Women's	★
Herbalife Multivitamin Complex	★★
Highland Laboratories (see Mt. Angel Vitamin Company)	
Hillestad Pharmaceuticals Sterling	★★★
Hillestad Summit Gold	★★½
Hillestad Summit Gold Special Formula	★★★
Hillestad Summit MAX	★★★
Immunotec Research Vitamin and Mineral Supplement	★★★½
Immuvit Plus Q10	½
Innate Response Formulas Food Multi II	★½
Innate Response Formulas Food Multi III BioMax	★★
Innate Response Formulas Food Multi IV	★★
Innate Response Formulas Maximum Food	★½
Innate Response Formulas Men Over 40	★★½
Innate Response Formulas Men over 40 One Daily	★½
Innate Response Formulas One Daily	★½
Innate Response Formulas One Daily Cap	★★½
Innate Response Formulas One Daily without Iron	★½
Innate Response Formulas Women Over 40	★★
Innate Response Formulas Women Over 40 One Daily	★½
Innate Response Formulas Women's Multi	★★
Innate Response Formulas Women's One Daily	★
Integrative Therapeutics Clinical Nutrients 45-Plus Women	★★★★½
Integrative Therapeutics Clinical Nutrients 50-Plus Men	★★★★½
Integrative Therapeutics Clinical Nutrients for Men	★★★★½
Integrative Therapeutics Clinical Nutrients for Women	★★★★½
Integrative Therapeutics Maximum Blue	★★★★
Integrative Therapeutics Mega MultiVitamin Powder Mix	★★★½
Integrative Therapeutics Multiplex-1 with Iron	★★★★
Integrative Therapeutics Multiplex-1 without Iron	★★★★½
Integrative Therapeutics Multiplex-2 with Iron	★★★★
Integrative Therapeutics Multiplex-2 without Iron	★★★★
Integrative Therapeutics NutriVitamin Enzyme Complex	★★★★½
Integrative Therapeutics NutriVitamin Enzyme Complex without Iron	★★★★
Integrative Therapeutics Spectrient	★★★½
Integrative Therapeutics Spectrient without Iron	★★★
Integrative Therapeutics Spectrum 2C with Iron	★★★
Integrative Therapeutics Spectrum 2C without Iron	★★★★½
Integrative Therapeutics Total Formula 2	★★★½
Integrative Therapeutics Total Formula 3 Advanced No Iron	★★★½
Intensive Nutrition Mega-VM	★★★★½
Intensive Nutrition Multi-VM	★★★★
Irwin Naturals Angel Multi	★★★½
Irwin Naturals Men's Living Green Liquid-Gel Multi	★★★½
Irwin Naturals Only One Liquid-Gel Multi	★★
Irwin Naturals Only One Liquid-Gel Multi without Iron	★★★½
Irwin Naturals Women's Living Green Liquid-Gel Multi	★★★½
Isagenix Essentials For Men	★★★½
Isagenix Essentials For Women	★★★½
Isotonix Multivitamin	★★★½
It Works! It's Vital Core Nutrition	★★★½
Jarrow Formulas Multi 1-to-3 (with Lutein)	★★★★
Jarrow Formulas Women's Multi	★★★★
JD Premium MVX Daily	★★★★★
Jean-Marc Brunet (see Le Naturiste)	
Jeunesse (see Nutrigen)	
KAL Enhanced 75	★★★½
KAL Enhanced Energy	★★★★
KAL Enhanced Energy Supreme Iron Free	★★★★½
KAL High Potency Soft Multiple	★★★

Manufacturer & Product Name	Rating
KAL High Potency Soft Multiple Iron Free	★★★½
KAL Mega Vita-Min	★★★
KAL Multi-Active Iron Free	★★★★
KAL Multi-Four +	★★★★
KAL Multi-Max 1	★★½
KAL Multi-Max 1 50+ Sustained Release	★★★½
KAL Multi-Max 1 for Men	★★★
KAL Multi-Max 1 for Women Sustained Release	★★½
KAL Multi-Max 1 Iron Free	★★★
Karuna Maxxum 1	★★★★½
Karuna Maxxum 2	★★★★½
Karuna Maxxum 3	★★★★½
Karuna Maxxum 4	★★★★½
Karuna Maxxum Basic	★★★
Kirkland Signature Daily Multi	★
Kirkland Signature Mature Multi	★½
Kirkland Signature Premium Performance Multi	★½
Kirkman EveryDay	★½
Kirkman Spectrum Complete II	★★½
Leader Mega Multivitamin for Men	★★
Leader Mega Multivitamin for Women	★★½
Leader One Daily Men's Health	★
Leader One Daily Plus Iron	½
Leader One Daily Weight Control	★½
Leader One Daily Women's	½
Levity+Plus Multivitamin for Women	★★★
Life Solutions Super MultiVitamins and Minerals	★★★
LifeExtension LifeExtension Mix	★★★★★
LifeExtension LifeExtension Mix Extra Niacin Without Copper	★★★★★
LifeExtension LifeExtension Mix With Extra Niacin	★★★★★
LifeExtension LifeExtension Mix Without Copper	★★★★★
LifeExtension One-Per-Day	★★★★½
LifeExtension Two-Per-Day	★★★★½
LifeGive Men's Formula	★½
LifeGive Women's Formula	★½
Life-Line Vitamin Multimineral	★★½
Lifeplus Daily BioBasics	★★★
Lifeplus TVM-Plus	★★★
LifeScript Daily Essentials	★½
LifeSource Men's Superior	★★★★
LifeSource Multi Vitamin & Minerals	★★★½
LifeSource Women's Superior	★★★½
Lifetime Fitness Men's Performance Daily AM/PM	★★★★½
Lifetime Fitness Women's Performance Daily AM/PM	★★★★½
LifeTime Soft Gel	★★★
Liquid Health Complete Multiple	★★
LiquiMax Complete Nutrition	★
Mannatech PhytoMatrix	★½
Martha Stewart Essentials	★★
Mason Natural Daily Multiple Vitamins with Minerals	★
Mason Natural Super Multiple Iron Free	★★
Mason Natural VitaTRUM	½
Matol Mega Vitamins	★★½
Mauves (see Trophic)	
Max International Max N-Fuze	★★
Maxi Health Maxi Longevity	★★★½
Maxi Health Maxicaps	★★★
Maxi Health Maxivite Complete	★★½
Maxi Health Supreme	★★★★½
Maxi Vision Whole Body Formula	★★★★½
Maximized Living Women's Multi	★★½
Maximum Human Performance Activite	★★★
Maxion Max Multi	★★
MBi Bio-Naturalvite	★★
MD Healthline Advanced Green Multi	½
MD's Choice Complete Formula	★★★½
MD's Choice Complete Formula for Mature Women	★★★★½
MD's Choice Complete Formula for Men	★★★★½
MD's Choice Complete Formula for Young Women	★★★★½
MD's Choice Complete Liquid Formula	★★★½
MegaFood Lifestyle	★★
MegaFood Lifestyle One Daily	½
MegaFood Men over 40	★★½
MegaFood Men Over 40 One Daily	★½
MegaFood Men's	★★

Manufacturer & Product Name	Rating
MegaFood Men's One Daily	★½
MegaFood One Daily	★½
MegaFood Optimum Foods	★½
MegaFood Women Over 40	★★
MegaFood Women Over 40 One Daily	★½
MegaFood Women's	★★
MegaFood Women's One Daily	★
Melaleuca Vitality Men's	★★½
Melaleuca Vitality Women's	★★
Member's Mark Complete Multi	½
Metabolic Maintenance Basic Maintenance	★★
Metabolic Maintenance Basic Maintenance Plus Vitamin D	★★½
Metagenics Multigenics	★★★★
Metagenics Multigenics Chewable	★★
Metagenics Multigenics Intensive Care	★★★★½
Metagenics Multigenics Intensive Care without Iron	★★★★½
Metagenics Multigenics Powder	★★★½
Metagenics Multigenics without Iron	★★★★½
Metagenics PhytoMulti	★★★
Metagenics PhytoMulti with Iron	★★★
Michael's Naturopathic Programs For Men	★★★½
Michael's Naturopathic Programs For Women	★★★
Miracle 2000 Total Body Nutrition	★★★½
More Than a Multiple Iron-Free / Vegetarian Formula	★★★
More Than a Multiple Multivitamin for Men	★★★★
More than a Multiple Multivitamin for Women	★★★½
More Than a Multiple Multivitamin Formula	★★★★
Mountain Naturals of Vermont Daily Best	★★★
Mountain Naturals of Vermont Superior Care without Copper & Iron	★★★★½
Mountain Peak Nutritionals Ultra High	★★★★
MRM Beyond Basics	★★★½
Mt. Angel Vitamin Company Men's 50+	★★★★
Mt. Angel Vitamin Company One Good Multi	★★★½
Mt. Angel Vitamin Company Simply 4 Energy	★★★★
Mt. Angel Vitamin Company Women's 50+	★★★★
MultiSure (see Webber Naturals)	
Myadec Multivitamin Multimineral Supplement	★
N.F. Formulas (see Integrative Therapeutics)	

Manufacturer & Product Name	Rating
Natrol My Favorite Multiple	★★½
Natrol My Favorite Multiple Energizer	★★
Natrol My Favorite Multiple for Women	★★★
Natrol My Favorite Multiple Iron Free	★★★½
Natrol My Favorite Multiple Prime	★★
Natrol My Favorite Multiple Prime 50+	★★★½
Natrol My Favorite Multiple Take One	★★½
Natural Factors Men's 50+ MultiStart	★★★★
Natural Factors Men's MultiStart	★★★★½
Natural Factors Women's MultiStart	★★★★
Natural Factors Women's Plus MultiStart	★★★★½
Natural Vitality Organic Life Vitamins	★★★
Naturally Preferred Life Multi Complete	★
Naturally Preferred Men's Multi	★½
Naturally Preferred One Daily Multi	★½
Naturally Preferred One Daily Multi Iron Free	★½
Naturally Preferred Vita-Max	★★★
Naturally Preferred Women's Multi	★
Nature Made Multi Complete Liquid Softgel	★
Nature Made Multi Complete Tablet	★½
Nature Made Multi for Her	★
Nature Made Multi for Her 50+	★½
Nature Made Multi for Him 50+	★★
Nature's Answer Multi-Daily	★½
Nature's Answer Platinum Liquid Multiple Vitamin & Mineral	★★½
Nature's Best A to Z	★
Nature's Best Multi-Max 50 Plus	★★
Nature's Best Multi-Max Complete	★★★
Nature's Blend Multi-Vitamin with Minerals	½
Nature's Bounty Multi-Day Plus Minerals	½
Nature's Bounty Multi-Day Women's	★
Nature's Bounty Your Life Adult Gummies	★½
Nature's Bounty Your Life Men's 45+	★½
Nature's Bounty Your Life Women's 45+	★
Nature's Life Antioxidant Soft Multi	★★★★
Nature's Life E-Z Vite Multiple	★½
Nature's Life Great Greens Multi	★★★½
Nature's Life Green-Pro 96 Multi	★★
Nature's Life One Daily	★★★½
Nature's Life Soft Gelatin Multiple	★★★
Nature's Life Vegan Super Mega Vite	★★★

Manufacturer & Product Name	Rating
Nature's Plus Ageless Men's Multi	★★★★
Nature's Plus Ageless Women's Multi	★★★½
Nature's Plus Especially Yours	★★★
Nature's Plus Mega Force	★★★★
Nature's Plus Source of Life	★★★½
Nature's Plus Source of Life (no iron)	★★★★
Nature's Plus Source of Life Adult's Chewable	★★★
Nature's Plus Source of Life Gold	★★★★½
Nature's Plus Source of Life Green and Red	★★★★
Nature's Plus Source of Life Men	★★★★
Nature's Plus Source of Life Men Liquid	★★★½
Nature's Plus Source of Life Red	★★★★
Nature's Plus Source of Life Women	★★★½
Nature's Plus Source of Life Women Liquid	★★★½
Nature's Plus Ultra Source of Life	★★★½
Nature's Plus Ultra Source of Life No Iron	★★★★
Nature's Secret Women's 73 Nutrient Soft-Gel Multi	★★½
Nature's Sunshine Super Supplemental	★★★
Nature's Way Alive! Energy 50+	★★
Nature's Way Alive! Liquid Multi	★★★½
Nature's Way Alive! Men's Energy	★★
Nature's Way Alive! Men's Multi	★★★★
Nature's Way Alive! Men's Ultra Potency	★★★½
Nature's Way Alive! Multi-Vitamin	★★★½
Nature's Way Alive! Multi-Vitamin (No Iron Added)	★★★★½
Nature's Way Alive! Multi-Vitamin Ultra Potency	★★★
Nature's Way Alive! Women's Energy	★½
Nature's Way Alive! Women's Multi	★★★★
New Chapter every MAN	★★
New Chapter Every Man II	★★★½
New Chapter Every Man's One Daily	★★
New Chapter Every Man's One Daily 40+	★★
New Chapter Every Woman	★★
New Chapter Every Woman II	★★★½
New Chapter Every Woman's One Daily	★★
New Chapter Every Woman's One Daily 40+	★★
New Chapter Only One	★★
New Chapter Perfect Calm	★★★½
New Chapter Perfect Energy	★★★½
New Chapter Perfect Immune	★★

Manufacturer & Product Name	Rating
New Chapter Tiny Tabs	★★
Neways Maximol Solutions	½
Nikken Mega Daily 4 for Men	★★½
Nikken Mega Daily 4 for Women	★★½
NorthStar Nutritionals RegeneCell	★★★★★
NorthStar Nutritionals Ultimate Daily Support	★★★★½
NOW Adam	★★★★
NOW Adam Superior	★★★★
NOW Daily Vits	★
NOW Eve	★★★★
NOW Liquid Multi Gels	★★★
NOW Special One	★★
NOW Special Two	★★★★
NOW Vit-Min 100	★★★½
NOW Vit-Min 75+	★★★½
Nutra Perfect Dentra Perfect	★★
Nutra Perfect VitaPerfect	★★★½
Nutra Therapeutics (see Adëeva)	
Nutraceutical Research Institute Mega 2	★★★
Nutralife Ultra Daily	★★★½
NutraMetrix Isotonix with Iron	★★
NutraOrigin Men & Women	★★★
NutraOrigin Men's	★★★
NutraOrigin Women's	★★★½
NutriCology Complete Immune	★★★★½
NutriCology Multi-Vi-Min	★★
NutriCology Multi-Vi-Min without Copper and Iron	★★
NutriCology MVM-A	★★★
NutriCology WomanPrime	★★
Nutriex Basic	★★★★
Nutriex Health	★★★★½
NutriGen AM & PM Essentials	★★
Nutrilite Daily	★½
Nutrilite Daily Free Multivitamin Multimineral	★½
Nutrina Vitamax Powder	★★★
Nutrina Vitamax Tablets	★★
Nutri-Supreme Research Active 50 Plus	★★★★
Nutri-Supreme Research ltra Multi 2	★★★½
Nutri-Supreme Research Muilti 1	★★★★½
Nutri-Supreme Research Multi-Vitamins Once Daily	★★★

Manufacturer & Product Name	Rating
Nutrition Dynamics Optimum Health Essentials	★★★★½
Nutrition Now MultiVites	★½
NuTriVene Adult Daily	★★★★½
NuTriVene Full Spectrum Formula	★★★★
Nutri-West Core Level Health Reserve	★
Nutri-West Multi Complex	★½
Nutri-West MultiBalance For Men	★★½
Nutri-West MultiBalance For Women	★★½
O'Brien Pharmacy Optimal Daily Allowance	★★★★½
Ola Loa Energy Daily Multi	★★★½
Olympian Labs Vita-Vitamin	★★★½
Omninutrition Omni IV	★
One A Day Energy	★
One A Day Menopause Formula	★½
One A Day Men's 50+ Advantage	★½
One A Day Men's Health Formula	★½
One A Day Men's Pro Edge	★½
One A Day VitaCraves	★
One A Day Women's	★
One A Day Women's 50+ Advantage	★½
One A Day Women's Active Metabolism	★
One A Day Women's Petites	★
One A Day Women's plus Healthy Skin Support	★
OneSource Men's	★★★½
OneSource Women's	★★★
Only Natural For Women Only	★½
Only Natural Mega Multi Energizer	★★★★
Optimox Androvite	★★★★
Optimox Gynovite Plus	★★★
Optimox Optivite P.M.T.	★★★★
Optimum Nutrition Opti-Men	★★★½
Optimum Nutrition Opti-Women	★★½
Oregon Health Multi-Guard	★★★★★
Orenda International All in One Female	★★★½
Orenda International All in One Male	★★★½
Orenda International All in One Young & Active	★★★★
Ortho Molecular Products Alpha Base with Iron	★★★★½
Ortho Molecular Products Alpha Base without Iron	★★★★½
Ortho Molecular Products Mitocore	★★★½

Manufacturer & Product Name	Rating
OxyLife Liquid Oxy-Gold	★★★
Perque Perque 2 Life Guard	★★★★
Pharmanex Life Essentials	★★
Pharmanex Vitox	★★½
PharmAssure Complete Multivite	★½
PharmAssure Men's Biomultiple	★★★
PharmAssure Women's Biomultiple	★★
Physician Formulas MultiVit Rx	★★★★½
Physician's Preference Dr. Hotze's Energy Formula	★★★★½
Pioneer 1 + 1 Vitamin Mineral	★★★★
Pioneer 1 + Vitamin Mineral	★★★½
Pioneer 1 + Vitamin Mineral Iron Free	★★★★
Pioneer Chewable	★★★★
Pioneer Chewable Iron Free	★★★½
Pioneer Vitamin Mineral	★★★★½
Platinum Performance Platinum Multi-Vitamin & Mineral Formula	★★
Poliquin Complete Multi 2.0	★★★★
Poliquin Complete Multi 2.0 Iron Free	★★★★½
Poliquin Multi Intense	★★★★½
Poliquin Multi Intense Iron Free	★★★★½
Poliquin Über Nutrients	★★★
Poliquin Über Nutrients Iron Free	★★★
Pro Grade VGF 25+ for Men	★★★½
Pro Grade VGF 25+ for Women	★★★½
Pro Health Super Multiple II	★★★★
Pro Image Pro Vitamin Complete	★
Pro-Caps Laboratories Essential 1	★★★½
ProThera MultiThera 1	★★★★½
ProThera MultiThera 2	★★★★½
ProThera VitaTab Chewable	★★★½
ProThera VitaTab VitaPrime	★★★★½
ProThera VitaTab VitaPrime Capsules	★★★½
Pure Encapsulations Men's Nutrients	★★★★½
Pure Encapsulations Multi t/d	★★★★½
Pure Encapsulations Nutrient 950	★★★★★
Pure Encapsulations O.N.E. Multivitamin	★★★★½
Pure Encapsulations PureFood Nutrients	★½
Pure Encapsulations Women's Nutrients	★★★★½
Pure Essence Labs LifeEssence Powder	★★★★½
Pure Essence Labs LifeEssence Vegetarian Formula	★★★★½

Manufacturer & Product Name	Rating
Pure Essence Labs LifeEssence Women's Formula	★★★★½
Pure Essence Labs Longevity Men's Formula	★★★★½
Pure Essence Labs Longevity Women's Formula	★★★★½
Pure Essence Labs One 'n' Only	★★★½
Pure Essence Labs One 'n' Only Men's Formula	★★★★
Pure Essence Labs One 'n' Only Women's Formula	★★★
Pure Synergy Organic Multi Vita-Min	★★½
Pure Synergy Organic Vita-Min-Herb for Men	★★★★
Pure Synergy Organic Vita-Min-Herb for Women	★★★★
Puritan's Pride ABC Plus	½
Puritan's Pride Mega Vita-Min	★★★
Puritan's Pride One Daily Men's	★½
Puritan's Pride Vita-Min Complete Formula #1	★
Puritan's Pride Women's One Daily	★
Purity Products Perfect Multi	★★★★½
Purity Products Perfect Multi Essentials	★★★★
Purity Products Perfect Multi Focus Formula	★★★★
Purity Products Perfect Multi Liquid	★★★½
Purity Products Perfect Multi Super Greens	★★★★½
Purpose (See Creating Wellness)	
QCI Nutritionals Daily Preventive #1	★★★★½
Rainbow Light 50+ Mini-Tab	★★★
Rainbow Light Active Senior	★★★
Rainbow Light Advanced Nutritional System	★★★★½
Rainbow Light Advanced Nutritional System Iron-Free	★★★★½
Rainbow Light Certified Organics Men's Multivitamin	★★
Rainbow Light Certified Organics Women's Multivitamin	★★
Rainbow Light Complete Nutritional System	★★★★½
Rainbow Light Complete Nutritional System Iron-Free	★★★★
Rainbow Light Energizer One	★★★
Rainbow Light Just Once	★★
Rainbow Light Just Once Iron-Free	★★
Rainbow Light Men's One	★★★½
Rainbow Light Performance Energy for Men	★★★

Manufacturer & Product Name	Rating
Rainbow Light RejuvenAge 40+	★★★★½
Rainbow Light Women's Nutritional System	★★★★
Rainbow Light Women's One	★★½
Ray & Terry's Total Care Daily Formula	★★★½
Ray & Terry's Two-a-Day	★★★½
Real Advantage Nutrients Ultimate Daily Support	★★★★½
Rejuvenation Science Maximum Vitality	★★★★★
Reliv Classic	★½
Reliv Now	★★
Reserveage Organics Vibrance	★★★★
Restorage Professional for Men & Women	★½
Revival Firm Foundation Multivitamin Multimineral 100	★★
Rexall (see Sundown Naturals)	
R-Garden Daily Complete	★★★★
Rite Aid Central-Vite	½
Rite Aid Central-Vite Cardio	★
Rite Aid Central-Vite Men's Mature	★½
Rite Aid Central-Vite Performance	★
Rite Aid Central-Vite Select	★
Rite Aid Central-Vite Women's Mature	★½
Rite Aid One Daily Energy Formula	★
Rite Aid One Daily Men's Multi	★
Rite Aid One Daily Women's	½
Rite Aid One Daily Women's 50+	★½
Rite Aid ResurgenC	★
Rite Aid Whole Source Men	★★
Rite Aid Whole Source Women	★½
Rx Vitamins ReVitalize	★★★★
Safeway Active Performance	★
Safeway Century	★
Safeway Century Ultimate Men's	★
Safeway Century Ultimate Women's	★
Safeway Complete for Adults 50+	★
Safeway One Daily Men's 50+ Advanced	★½
Safeway One Daily Men's Health Formula	★
Safeway Ultimate Women's 50+	★½
Safeway Women's 50+	★½
SAN Multi Nutrient Formula Basic	★★★★
SAN Multi Nutrient Formula Gold	★★★★½
SAN Multi Nutrient Formula Original	★★★★½
SAN Multi Nutrient Formula Plus	★★★★½

Manufacturer & Product Name	Rating
Saturn Supplements Vitaplex	★½
Schiff Single Day	★★★
Schiff Vegetarian Multiple	★½
Schwartz Laboratories VitaPlex	★★★★
Schwarzbein Institute Ultra Preventive III (Capsules)	★★★½
Schwarzbein Principle Ultra Preventive III (Tablets)	★★★★½
Sentinel Mega Multi	★★★
Sentinel One Daily	½
Sentinel One Daily with Iron	½
Sentinel Sentivites Senior	★
Sentinel Therra M	★
Shaklee CitriBoost	★½
Shaklee Vita-Lea Gold Vitamin K	★★½
Shaklee Vita-Lea Gold without Vitamin K	★★½
Shaklee Vita-Lea Iron Formula	★★
Shaklee Vita-Lea without Iron Formula	★★½
Solaray Iron Free Spectro	★★★
Solaray Men's Golden	★★★½
Solaray Multi-Vita Mega-Mineral	★★★½
Solaray Once Daily High Energy	★★½
Solaray Provide	★★★½
Solaray Spectro	★★½
Solaray Spectro 3	★★★
Solaray Spectro 3 Iron Free	★★★½
Solaray Spectro 50-Plus	★★★½
Solaray Spectro Man	★★½
Solaray Spectro Vegetarian	★★½
Solaray Spectro Woman	★★½
Solaray Three Daily Super Energy	★★★★
Solaray Three Daily Super Energy Iron Free	★★★★
Solaray Twice Daily Multi Energy	★★★
Solaray Twice Daily Multi Energy Iron Free	★★★½
Solaray VitaPrime For Men	★★★½
Solaray VitaPrime For Women	★★★½
Solaray Women's Golden	★★★½
Solgar Earth Source Multi-Nutrient	★★★½
Solgar Female Multiple	★★★★
Solgar Formula VM-75	★★★
Solgar Formula VM-75 Iron-Free	★★★
Solgar Male Multiple	★★★★½
Source Naturals Advanced One (No Iron)	★★★★
Source Naturals Advanced One (with Iron)	★★★½
Source Naturals Élan Vitàl Multiple	★★★★½
Source Naturals Life Force Green Multiple	★★★★½
Source Naturals Life Force Multiple	★★★★½
Source Naturals Life Force Vegan	★★★★★
Source Naturals Life Force Vegan No Iron	★★★★★
Source Naturals Mega-One	★★★
Source Naturals Mega-One No Iron	★★★½
Source Naturals Men's Life Force Multiple	★★★★★
Source Naturals Ultra Multiple	★★★
Source Naturals Wellness Multiple	★★★½
Source Naturals Women's Life Force	★★★★★
Source Naturals Women's Life Force Multiple, No Iron	★★★★★
Spring Valley Adult Gummy Multivitamin	½
Spring Valley Ultra Multivitamin For Women	★★★
Standard Process Catalyn	½
STS Fit Man Multi	★★★½
STS Fit Woman Multi	★★★½
Sundown Naturals Adult Multivitamin Gummies	★½
Sundown Naturals Complete Daily	★
Sundown Naturals Complete Women's	★½
Sundown Naturals Daily	½
Sundown Naturals SunVite	★
Sundown Naturals SunVite Active Adults 50+	★
Sundown Naturals Whole Food Multivitamin	★★½
Super Nutrition Men's Blend	★★★★½
Super Nutrition Perfect Family	★★★★½
Super Nutrition Super Immune Multi Vitamin	★★★★★
Super Nutrition Women's Blend	★★★★½
Swanson Active One with Iron	★★
Swanson Active One without Iron	★★½
Swanson Active One without Iron Mini-Tabs	★★★
Swanson All-Day Complete for Seniors	★★★★
Swanson Century Formula with Iron	★
Swanson Century Formula without Iron	★½
Swanson Daily Multi-Vitamin & Mineral	★★
Swanson Geromulti without Iron	★½
Swanson High Potency Softgel Iron Free	★★★★½
Swanson Jack LaLanne Vita-Lanne Liquid	★★★
Swanson Longevital	★★★★★

Manufacturer & Product Name	Rating
Swanson Men's Prime Multi	★★
Swanson Vital Multi for Men	★★½
Swanson Vital Multi for Women	★★½
Swanson Whole Food Multi without Iron	★★★½
Swanson Women's Prime Multi	★★
The Results Company (see Vitamost)	
The Synergy Company (see Pure Synergy)	
Theragran-M Advanced	★
Theragran-M Advanced 50 Plus	★
Theragran-M Premier	★½
Theragran-M Premier 50 Plus	★★
Theralogix 50+ Companion Women's Multivitamin	★½
Theralogix Essentia Women's Multivitamin	★★
Thompson Adult-Plex	★★★½
Thompson All-In-One	★½
Thompson Coach's Formula	★★½
Thompson Mega 80	★★½
Thompson Multi Formula For Women	★
Thompson Multi Vitamins With Minerals	★½
Thompson Nuplex	★½
Thorne Research Al's Formula	★★★★
Thorne Research Basic Nutrients V	★★★★★
Thorne Research Extra Nutrients	★★★★
Thorne Research Meta-Fem	★★★★★½
Thorne Research Nutri-Fem	★★★★★
To Your Health Liquid Vitamins	★★★★½
Trace Minerals Research Liquid Multi Vita-Mineral	★★★
Trace Minerals Research Liquimins Maxi Multi	★★
Trader Joe's Men's Once Daily	★★★
Trader Joe's Multi Vitamin & Mineral Antioxidant	★★
Trader Joe's Women's Once Daily	★★★½
TriVita VitaDaily AM Formula & PM Formula	★★★
TriVita Wellavoh for Men AM Formula & PM Formula	★★★½
TriVita Wellavoh for Women AM Formula & PM Formula	★★★
Tropical Oasis Multiple Vitamin Mineral for Adults	★
True Essentials Adult Chewable	★½
True Essentials Everyday Essentials	★★★½

Manufacturer & Product Name	Rating
True Essentials Men's Everyday	★★★
True Essentials Women's Everyday	★★★
True Essentials Women's Gold	★★★
Truestar Health TrueBasics Solo	★★★★★ (grey)
Twinlab Allergy Multi Caps	★★★½
Twinlab Daily One Caps With Iron	★★½
Twinlab Daily One Caps Without Iron	★★½
Twinlab Daily Two Caps with Iron	★★★
Twinlab Daily Two Caps without iron	★★★½
Twinlab Dualtabs	★★★½
Twinlab Mega 6	★★★½
Twinlab Women's Ultra Daily	★★★½
Ultimate Nutrition Daily Complete Formula	★★★★
Ultimate Nutrition Super Complete Formula	★★★★½
Unicity Core Health Basics	★½
Univera MultiVitamin	★★
Universal Formulas Quint-Essence	★★★½
Up & Up Adults' Multivitamin/Multimineral	★
Up & Up Men's Daily	★½
Up & Up Multivitamin/Multimineral	★
Up & Up Women's Daily	★
Up &Up Multivitamin/Multimineral Adults 50+	★
Usana Health Sciences Essentials _Editor's Choice Award_	★★★★★ (grey)
Usana Health Sciences Essentials Kosher	★★★★½
Växa Daily Essentials	★½
VegLife MultiVeg Energy	★★★
VegLife MultiVeg Energy Iron Free	★★★½
VegLife SpectroVeg High Energy	★★½
VegLife Vegan One	★★½
VegLife Vegan One Iron Free	★★½
Visalus Multi Mineral & Vitamin	★★½
Vita Springs Anti-Aging Multi-Vitamins	★½
Vitacost Men's 50 Plus	★★★½
Vitacost Synergy 3000	★★★★½
Vitacost Synergy Basic	★★★★½
Vitacost Synergy Complete	★★★★
Vitacost Synergy Men's	★★★★½
Vitacost Synergy NeroPower	★★★★½
Vitacost Synergy Viva! No Added Iron	★★★★½
Vitacost Synergy Viva! with Iron	★★★★½
Vitacost Synergy Women's	★★★★½

Manufacturer & Product Name	Rating
Vitacost Synergy Women's with Iron	★★★★½
Vitacost The Woman	★★★★
Vitacost Women's 50 Plus	★★★
VitaFusion Men's	★½
VitaFusion MultiVites	★½
VitaFusion MultiVites Sour	★½
VitaFusion Women's	★½
Vital Nutrients Minimal and Essential	★★★★
Vital Nutrients Multi-Nutrients 2	★★★★
Vital Nutrients Multi-Nutrients 3	★★★★
Vital Nutrients Multi-Nutrients 4	★★★★
Vital Nutrients Multi-Nutrients 5	★★★★
Vital Nutrients Multi-Nutrients Veg	★★★★
Vital Nutrients Multi-Nutrients with Iron and Iodine	★★★½
Vital Nutrients Vital Clear	★★★★
VitaLabs Mega-2	★★½
Vitalert Energy Multi	★★
Vitality Men's Multi	★★
Vitality Multivite	★★½
Vitality Women's Multi	★★
Vitamark Primalux	★★★
VitaMedica Multi-Vitamin & Mineral	★★★★
Vitamin Code (see Garden of Life)	
Vitamin Power Advanced Multi-Vites & Mins	★
Vitamin Power Complete Men's Multiple	★★½
Vitamin Power Mega Multiple 85	★★
Vitamin Power Power Source 100	★★★
Vitamin Power Super Vite	★★
Vitamin Power Ultra Multi 90 Plus	★★★
Vitamin Research Products Extend Core	★★★★½
Vitamin Research Products Extend Liquid	★★★★
Vitamin Research Products Extend One	★★★★½
Vitamin Research Products Extend Plus	★★★★½
Vitamin Research Products Extend Ultra	★★★★½
Vitamin Research Products Optimum Protection	★★★★
Vitamin Research Products Optimum Silver	★★★★½
Vitamin Research Products Women's Essentials	★★★★
Vitamin Shoppe Especially for Men	★★★½
Vitamin Shoppe K Free Multi	★★★
Vitamin Shoppe Multi Vitamin & Mineral Powder	★★★★

Manufacturer & Product Name	Rating
Vitamin Shoppe Nutri-100 No Iron	★★★★½
Vitamin Shoppe One Daily	★★
Vitamin Shoppe One Daily with Lutein & Lycopene	★★½
Vitamin Shoppe One Daily with Lutein & Lycopene No Iron	★★½
Vitamin Shoppe One Daily without Iron	★★★½
Vitamin Shoppe Ultimate Man	★★★★
Vitamin Shoppe Ultimate Man 50+	★★★★½
Vitamin Shoppe Ultimate Man Gold	★★★★½
Vitamin Shoppe Ultimate Woman	★★★★
Vitamin Shoppe Ultimate Woman 50+	★★★★
Vitamin Shoppe Ultimate Woman Gold	★★★★½
Vitamin Shoppe Ultimate Woman Gold No Iron	★★★★½
Vitamin Shoppe Ultimate Woman No Iron	★★★★½
Vitamin Shoppe Ultimate Woman Sustained Release	★★★★
Vitamin Shoppe Whole Food Men's One Daily	★
Vitamin Shoppe Whole Food Women's One Daily	★
Vitamin World Mega Vita-Gel	★★★½
Vitamin World Mega Vita-Min	★★★½
Vitamin World Mega Vita-Min Adult Chewable	★★½
Vitaminol (see Le Naturiste)	
Vitamins Direct Time Fighters for Men	★★★★½
Vitamost Prime	★★★★★½
Vitanica Mid-Life Symmetry	★★★★½
Vitanica Women's Symmetry	★★★★½
Vitapril	★★
VIVA DailyGuard	★★★
VIVA for Life	★★
Viva Vitamins Complete Multi Extra Strength	★★★½
Viva Vitamins Complete Multi Extra Strength Iron and Copper Free	★★★
Viva Vitamins Complete Multi Regular Strength	★★
Viva Vitamins Complete Multi Regular Strength Iron and Copper Free	★★
Viva Vitamins Complete Multi Ultra Strength	★★★
Viva Vitamins V.M.T. Extra Strength	★★★★
Viva Vitamins V.M.T. Regular Strength	★★★
Viva Vitamins VegiSource	★★★★½

MANUFACTURER & PRODUCT NAME	RATING
WALGREENS A THRU Z ACTIVE PERFORMANCE	★
WALGREENS A THRU Z SELECT ULTIMATE MEN'S	★½
WALGREENS A THRU Z SELECT ULTIMATE WOMEN'S	★½
WALGREENS A THRU Z ULTIMATE WOMEN'S	★
WALGREENS ADVANCED FORMULA A THRU Z	★
WALGREENS ADVANCED FORMULA A THRU Z SELECT ADULTS 50+	★½
WALGREENS ONE DAILY ENERGY	★
WALGREENS ONE DAILY FOR MEN	★
WALGREENS ONE DAILY FOR MEN 50+ ADVANCED	★½
WALGREENS ONE DAILY FOR WOMAN	★
WALGREENS ONE DAILY FOR WOMEN 50+ ADVANCED	★½
WALGREENS ONE DAILY HEALTHY WEIGHT	½
WATKINS DAILY VITAMIN	★★
WELLGENIX BALANCED ESSENTIALS	★★
WELLNESS INTERNATIONAL NETWORK PHYTO-VITE	★★½
WELLNESS RESOURCES DAILY ENERGY MULTIPLE VITAMIN	★★★★
WELLNESSPRO MULTIVITAMIN COMPLEX FOR MEN	★★
WELLNESSPRO MULTIVITAMIN COMPLEX FOR WOMEN	★★
WORLD ORGANIC LIQUI-VITE & LIQUI-MINS	★★½
XYMOGEN ACTIVNUTRIENTS	★★★½
XYMOGEN ACTIVNUTRIENTS WITHOUT IRON	★★★½
YOLI VITAMIN & MINERAL	★★★★
YOR HEALTH YOR ESSENTIAL VITAMIN	★★★★
YOUNG AGAIN ALL YOUR VITAMINS & ALL YOUR MINERALS	★★
YOUNG LIVING MASTER FORMULA HERS	★★★½
YOUNG LIVING MASTER FORMULA HIS	★★★★
YOUNGEVITY BEYOND TANGY TANGERINE	★★★½
YOUNGEVITY MAJESTIC EARTH TROPICAL PLUS	★★
YOUNGEVITY ULTIMATE CLASSIC	★★★★½
YOUNGEVITY ULTIMATE TANGY TANGERINE	★★★★½
ZAHLER MULTIMITE	★★★½
ZAHLER MULTIVITE	★★
ZEAL FOR LIFE WELLNESS FORMULA	★½
ZIQUIN MIND AND BODY TONIC	★★

BIBLIOGRAPHY

Chapter One References

(1) Forman HJ and Boveris A. "Superoxide radical and hydrogen peroxide in mitochondria." in: *Free Radicals in Biology* (vol 5), Pryor WA (ed), Academic Press, New York NY, 1982, 65-89.

(2) Hekimi S, Lapointe J, Wen Y. Taking a "good" look at free radicals in the aging process. Trends Cell Biol 2011;21:569-576.

(3) Harman D. Aging: a theory based on free radical and radiation chemistry. *J Gerontol* 1956;11:298-300

(4) Harman D. The biologic clock: the mitochondria? *J Am Geriatr Soc* 1972;20:145-147.

(5) West ES, Todd W, Mason HS and Van Bruggen JT. *Textbook of Biochemistry 4th edition*. The Macmillan Co., Toronto ON, 1970, 899-903.

(6) Davies K. "Oxidative stress, the paradox of aerobic life." *Biochemical Society Symposia* 1995, 61: 1-31.

(7) Harman D. "Free radical theory of aging: effect of free radical reaction inhibitors on the mortality rate of male LAF mice." *J Gerontol* 1968, 23(4): 476-482.

Chapter Two References

(1) Studer M, Briel M, Leimenstoll B, Glass TR, Bucher HC. Effect of different antilipidemic agents and diets on mortality: a systematic review. *Arch Intern Med* 2005;165:725-730.

(2) Ross R. Atherosclerosis is an inflammatory disease. *Am Heart J* 1999;138:S419-S420.

(3) Albert CM, Ma J, Rifai N, Stampfer MJ, Ridker PM. Prospective study of C-reactive protein, homocysteine, and plasma lipid levels as predictors of sudden cardiac death. *Circulation* 2002;105:2595-2599.

(4) Bermudez EA, Ridker PM. C-reactive protein, statins, and the primary prevention of atherosclerotic cardiovascular disease. *Prev Cardiol* 2002;5:42-46.

(5) Rifai N, Ridker PM. Inflammatory markers and coronary heart disease. *Curr Opin Lipidol* 2002;13:383-389.

(6) Gorman C, Park A. The Fires Within. Time February 23. 2004. Time Publishers. Ref Type: Magazine Article

(7) Jager A, van H, V, Kostense PJ et al. von Willebrand factor, C-reactive protein, and 5-year mortality in diabetic and nondiabetic subjects: the Hoorn Study. *Arterioscler Thromb Vasc Biol* 1999;19:3071-3078.

(8) Ridker PM, Cushman M, Stampfer MJ, Tracy RP, Hennekens CH. Inflammation, aspirin, and the risk of cardiovascular disease in apparently healthy men. *N Engl J Med* 1997;336:973-979.

(9) Ridker PM, Buring JE, Shih J, Matias M, Hennekens CH. Prospective study of C-reactive protein and the risk of future cardiovascular events among apparently healthy women. *Circulation* 1998;98:731-733.

(10) Libby P, Ridker PM, Maseri A. Inflammation and atherosclerosis. *Circulation* 2002;105:1135-1143.

(11) Packard CJ, O'Reilly DS, Caslake MJ et al. Lipoprotein-associated phospholipase A2 as an independent predictor of coronary heart disease. West of Scotland Coronary Prevention Study Group. *N Engl J Med* 2000;343:1148-1155.

(12) Ridker PM, Rifai N, Stampfer MJ, Hennekens CH. Plasma concentration of interleukin-6 and the risk of future myocardial infarction among apparently healthy men. *Circulation* 2000;101:1767-1772.

(13) Jialal I, Devaraj S. Inflammation and atherosclerosis: the value of the high-sensitivity C-reactive protein assay as a risk marker. *Am J Clin Pathol* 2001;116 Suppl:S108-S115.

(14) Zairis MN, Papadaki OA, Manousakis SJ et al. C-reactive protein and multiple complex coronary artery plaques in patients with primary unstable angina. *Atherosclerosis* 2002;164:355-359.

(15) Sears B. *The Anti-Inflammation Zone*. New York, NY: HaperCollins Publishers Inc., 2005.

(16) Pompl PN, Ho L, Bianchi M, McManus T, Qin W, Pasinetti GM. A therapeutic role for cyclooxygenase-2 inhibitors in a transgenic mouse model of amyotrophic lateral sclerosis. *FASEB J* 2003;17:725-727.

(17) Schmidt R, Schmidt H, Curb JD, Masaki K, White LR, Launer LJ. Early inflammation and dementia: a 25-year follow-up of the Honolulu-Asia Aging Study. *Ann Neurol* 2002;52:168-174.

(18) Pradhan AD, Ridker PM. Do atherosclerosis and type 2 diabetes share a common inflammatory basis? *Eur Heart J* 2002;23:831-834.

(19) Kurzweil R, Grossman T. *Fantastic Voyage: Live Long Enough to Live Forever.* New York, NY: Rodale, 2004.

(20) Floyd RA. Neuroinflammatory processes are important in neurodegenerative diseases: an hypothesis to explain the increased formation of reactive oxygen and nitrogen species as major factors involved in neurodegenerative disease development. *Free Radic Biol Med* 1999;26:1346-1355.

(21) Arden NK, Cooper C. Osteoporosis in patients with inflammatory bowel disease. *Gut* 2002;50:9-10.

(22) Inflammatory bowel disease and the risk of fracture.: 2002.

(23) Valentine JF, Sninsky CA. Prevention and treatment of osteoporosis in patients with inflammatory bowel disease. *Am J Gastroenterol* 1999;94:878-883.

(24) Chung YC, Chang YF. Serum interleukin-6 levels reflect the disease status of colorectal cancer. *J Surg Oncol* 2003;83:222-226.

(25) Erlinger TP, Platz EA, Rifai N, Helzlsouer KJ. C-reactive protein and the risk of incident colorectal cancer. *JAMA* 2004;291:585-590.

(26) Burskins CJ, Ristimaki A, Offerhaus GJ ea. Role of Cyclooxygenase-2 in the development and treatment of oesophageal adenocarcinoma. *Scand J Gastroenterol* 2003;239:87-93.

(27) Reddy BS, Tokumo K, Kulkarni N, Aligia C, Kelloff G. Inhibition of colon carcinogenesis by prostaglandin synthesis inhibitors and related compounds. *Carcinogenesis* 1992;13:1019-1023.

(28) Akhmedkhanov A, Toniolo P, Zeleniuch-Jacquotte A, Koenig KL, Shore RE. Aspirin and lung cancer in women. *Br J Cancer* 2002;87:49-53.

(29) Duenwald M. Body's Defender Goes on the Attack. *The New York Times* January 22, 2002.

(30) Sears B. The Cause and the Cure for Silent Inflammation. *The Anti-Inflammation Zone.* New York, NY: HaperCollins Publishers Inc.; 2005;21-30.

(31) Cunningham DS. Quenching the Flames of Inflammation. Life Extension , 27-34. 2004. Ref Type: Magazine Article

(32) Griffiths RJ, Pettipher ER, Koch K et al. Leukotriene B4 plays a critical role in the progression of collagen-induced arthritis. *Proc Natl Acad Sci U S A* 1995;92:517-521.

(33) Turner CR, Breslow R, Conklyn MJ et al. In vitro and in vivo effects of leukotriene B4 antagonism in a primate model of asthma. *J Clin Invest* 1996;97:381-387.

(34) Weringer EJ, Perry BD, Sawyer PS, Gilman SC, Showell HJ. Antagonizing leukotriene B4 receptors delays cardiac allograft rejection in mice. *Transplantation* 1999;67:808-815.

(35) Jiang Q, Elson-Schwab I, Courtemanche C, Ames BN. gamma-tocopherol and its major metabolite, in contrast to alpha-tocopherol, inhibit cyclooxygenase activity in macrophages and epithelial cells. *Proc Natl Acad Sci U S A* 2000;97:11494-11499.

(36) Jiang Q, Christen S, Shigenaga MK, Ames BN. gamma-tocopherol, the major form of vitamin E in the US diet, deserves more attention. *Am J Clin Nutr* 2001;74:714-722.

(37) Bengmark S. Curcumin, an atoxic antioxidant and natural NFkappaB, cyclooxygenase-2, lipooxygenase, and inducible nitric oxide synthase inhibitor: a shield against acute and chronic diseases. *JPEN J Parenter Enteral Nutr* 2006;30:45-51.

(38) Kurzweil R, Grossman T. Inflammation-the Latest "Smoking Gun". *Fantastic Voyage: Live Long Enough to Live Forever.* New York, NY: Rodale; 2004;160-171.

(39) Jenkins DJ, Kendall CW, Marchie A et al. Direct comparison of dietary portfolio vs statin on C-reactive protein. *Eur J Clin Nutr* 2005;59:851-860.

(40) Schmidt MA. *Smart Fats: How Dietary Fats and Oils affect Mental, Physical, and Emotional Intelligence.* Berkely, CA: Frog Ltd., 1997.

(41) Kelley VE, Ferretti A, Izui S, Strom TB. A fish oil diet rich in eicosapentaenoic acid reduces cyclooxygenase metabolites, and suppresses lupus in MRL-lpr mice. *J Immunol* 1985;134:1914-1919.

(42) Watanabe S, Katagiri K, Onozaki K et al. Dietary docosahexaenoic acid but not eicosapentaenoic acid suppresses lipopolysaccharide-induced interleukin-1 beta mRNA induction in mouse spleen leukocytes. *Prostaglandins Leukot Essent Fatty Acids* 2000;62:147-152.

(43) Murray MT. Essential Fatty Acid Supplementation. *Encyclopedia of Nutritional Supplements.* Rocklin, CA: Prima Health; 1996;249-278.

(44) Conner EM, Grisham MB. Inflammation, free radicals, and antioxidants. *Nutrition* 1996;12:274-277.

(45) Djordjevic VB. Free radicals in cell biology. *Int Rev Cytol* 2004;237:57-89.

(46) Rahman I. Oxidative stress, chromatin remodeling and gene transcription in inflammation and chronic lung diseases. *J Biochem Mol Biol* 2003;36:95-109.

(47) Winrow VR, Winyard PG, Morris CJ, Blake DR. Free radicals in inflammation: second messengers and mediators of tissue destruction. *Br Med Bull* 1993;49:506-522.

(48) Perricone N. The Inflammation-Aging-Disease-Obesity Connection. *The Perricone Weight-Loss Diet*. New York, NY: Ballantine Books; 2005;9-16.

(49) Goepp JG. What is Nuclear Factor kappa Beta? Life Extension July, 31-40. 2006. Ref Type: Magazine Article

(50) Ahn KS, Aggarwal BB. Transcription Factor NF-kB: A Sensor for Smoke and Stress Signals. *Ann NY Acad Sci* 2005;1056:218-233.

(51) Aggarwal BB, Shishodia S. Suppression of Nuclear Factor-kB Acivation Pathway by Spice-Derived Phytochemicals: Reasoning for Seasoning. *Ann NY Acad Sci* 2004;1030:434.

(52) Greenwell I. The Role of Inflammation in Chronic Disease. Life Extension Magazine Feb. 2001. Life Extension Media. Ref Type: Magazine Article

(53) Egan RW, Gale PH, Beveridge GC, Phillips GB, Marnett LJ. Radical scavenging as the mechanism for stimulation of prostaglandin cyclooxygenase and depression of inflammation by lipoic acid and sodium iodide. *Prostaglandins* 1978;16:861-869.

(54) Lee HA, Hughes DA. Alpha-lipoic acid modulates NF-kappaB activity in human monocytic cells by direct interaction with DNA. *Exp Gerontol* 2002;37:401-410.

(55) Ha H, Lee JH, Kim HN et al. alpha-Lipoic acid inhibits inflammatory bone resorption by suppressing prostaglandin E2 synthesis. *J Immunol* 2006;176:111-117.

(56) Burkart V, Koike T, Brenner HH, Imai Y, Kolb H. Dihydrolipoic acid protects pancreatic islet cells from inflammatory attack. *Agents Actions* 1993;38:60-65.

(57) Cho YS, Lee J, Lee TH et al. alpha-Lipoic acid inhibits airway inflammation and hyperresponsiveness in a mouse model of asthma. *J Allergy Clin Immunol* 2004;114:429-435.

(58) Grimble RF. Effect of antioxidative vitamins on immune function with clinical applications. *Int J Vitam Nutr Res* 1997;67:312-320.

(59) Majewicz J, Rimbach G, Proteggente AR, Lodge JK, Kraemer K, Minihane AM. Dietary vitamin C down-regulates inflammatory gene expression in apoE4 smokers. *Biochem Biophys Res Commun* 2005;338:951-955.

(60) Tahir M, Foley B, Pate G et al. Impact of vitamin E and C supplementation on serum adhesion molecules in chronic degenerative aortic stenosis: a randomized controlled trial. *Am Heart J* 2005;150:302-306.

(61) Majano PL, Garcia-Monzon C, Garcia-Trevijano ER et al. S-Adenosylmethionine modulates inducible nitric oxide synthase gene expression in rat liver and isolated hepatocytes. *J Hepatol* 2001;35:692-699.

Chapter Three References

(1) Marler JB, Wallin JR. Human Health, the Nutritional Quality of Harvested Food and Sustainable Farming Systems. *Nutrition Security Institute* [serial online] 2006; Accessed November 4, 2009.

(2) Thomas D. The mineral depletion of foods available to us as a nation (1940-2002)--a review of the 6th Edition of McCance and Widdowson. *Nutr Health* 2007;19:21-55.

(3) Farm Land Mineral Depletion. *Medical Missionary Press* [serial online] 2009; Accessed November 4, 2009.

(4) Horrigan L, Lawrence RS, Walker P. How sustainable agriculture can address the environmental and human health harms of industrial agriculture. *Environ Health Perspect* 2002;110:445-456.

(5) Lilburne LR, Hewitt AE, Sparling GP, Selvarajah N. Soil quality in New Zealand: policy and the science response. *J Environ Qual* 2002;31:1768-1773.

(6) McMichael AJ. Global environmental change and human health: new challenges to scientist and policy-maker. *J Public Health Policy* 1994;15:407-419.

(7) Boardman J, Shepheard ML, Walker E, Foster ID. Soil erosion and risk-assessment for on- and off-farm impacts: a test case using the Midhurst area, West Sussex, UK. *J Environ Manage* 2009;90:2578-2588.

(8) Griffin TS, Honeycutt CW. Effectiveness and efficacy of conservation options after potato harvest. *J Environ Qual* 2009;38:1627-1635.

(9) Gunderson PD. Biofuels and North American agriculture--implications for the health and safety of North American producers. *J Agromedicine* 2008;13:219-224.

(10) Liu YY, Ukita M, Imai T, Higuchi T. Recycling mineral nutrients to farmland via compost application. *Water Sci Technol* 2006;53:111-118.

(11)   Robert M. [Degradation of soil quality: health and environmental risks]. *Bull Acad Natl Med* 1997;181:21-40.

(12)   Davis DR, Epp MD, Riordan HD. Changes in USDA food composition data for 43 garden crops, 1950 to 1999. *J Am Coll Nutr* 2004;23:669-682.

(13)   Vegetables without Vitamins. Life Extension Foundation [March]. 2001. Ref Type: Magazine Article

(14)   Thomas D. A study on the mineral depletion of the foods available to us as a nation over the period 1940 to 1991. *Nutr Health* 2003;17:85-115.

(15)   Picard A. Today's fruits and vegetables lack yesterday's nutrition. *Globe and Mail* [serial online] 2002; Accessed November 4, 9 A.D.

(16)   Fan MS, Zhao FJ, Fairweather-Tait SJ, Poulton PR, Dunham SJ, McGrath SP. Evidence of decreasing mineral density in wheat grain over the last 160 years. *J Trace Elem Med Biol* 2008;22:315-324.

(17)   Hum M. untitled. *Institute for Optimum Nutrition* [serial online] 2006; Accessed November 3, 2014.

(18)   Karr M. Mineral Depletion in Soils. *longevitylibrary com* [serial online] 2009; Accessed November 4, 2009.

(19)   Drucker R. Depleted Soil and Compromised Food Sources: What You Can Do about It. *Nutrition Wellness* [serial online] 2006; Accessed May 11, 2009.

(20)   Soil Mineral Depletion: Can a Healthy diet be sufficient in today's world? *Physical Nutrition* [serial online] 2009; Available from: Botanica Medica. Accessed May 11, 2009.

(21)   Stockdale T. A speculative discussion of some problems arising from the use of ammonium nitrate fertiliser on acid soil. *Nutr Health* 1992;8:207-222.

(22)   Soil Depletion. *TJ Clark com* [serial online] 2006; Accessed November 4, 2009.

(23)   Ackerman LB. Overview of human exposure to dieldrin residues in the environment and current trends of residue levels in tissue. *Pestic Monit J* 1980;14:64-69.

(24)   Albers JM, Kreis IA, Liem AK, van ZP. Factors that influence the level of contamination of human milk with poly-chlorinated organic compounds. *Arch Environ Contam Toxicol* 1996;30:285-291.

(25)   Baillie-Hamilton PF. Chemical toxins: a hypothesis to explain the global obesity epidemic. *J Altern Complement Med* 2002;8:185-192.

(26)   Bharadwaj L, Dhami K, Schneberger D, Stevens M, Renaud C, Ali A. Altered gene expression in human hepatoma HepG2 cells exposed to low-level 2,4-dichlorophenoxyacetic acid and potassium nitrate. *Toxicol In Vitro* 2005;19:603-619.

(27)   Biscardi D, De FR, Feretti D et al. [Genotoxic effects of pesticide-treated vegetable extracts using the Allium cepa chromosome aberration and micronucleus tests]. *Ann Ig* 2003;15:1077-1084.

(28)   Carpy SA, Kobel W, Doe J. Health risk of low-dose pesticides mixtures: a review of the 1985-1998 literature on combination toxicology and health risk assessment. *J Toxicol Environ Health B Crit Rev* 2000;3:1-25.

(29)   Dougherty CP, Henricks HS, Reinert JC, Panyacosit L, Axelrad DA, Woodruff TJ. Dietary exposures to food contaminants across the United States. *Environ Res* 2000;84:170-185.

(30)   Grote K, Andrade AJ, Grande SW et al. Effects of peripubertal exposure to triphenyltin on female sexual development of the rat. *Toxicology* 2006;222:17-24.

(31)   Gupta PK. Pesticide exposure--Indian scene. *Toxicology* 2004;198:83-90.

(32)   Jiang QT, Lee TK, Chen K et al. Human health risk assessment of organochlorines associated with fish consumption in a coastal city in China. *Environ Pollut* 2005;136:155-165.

(33)   Katz JM, Winter CK. Comparison of pesticide exposure from consumption of domestic and imported fruits and vegetables. *Food Chem Toxicol* 2009;47:335-338.

(34)   Kawahara J, Yoshinaga J, Yanagisawa Y. Dietary exposure to organophosphorus pesticides for young children in Tokyo and neighboring area. *Sci Total Environ* 2007;378:263-268.

(35)   Luo Y, Zhang M. Multimedia transport and risk assessment of organophosphate pesticides and a case study in the northern San Joaquin Valley of California. *Chemosphere* 2009;75:969-978.

(36)   Moser VC, Simmons JE, Gennings C. Neurotoxicological interactions of a five-pesticide mixture in preweanling rats. *Toxicol Sci* 2006;92:235-245.

(37)   Nakata H, Kawazoe M, Arizono K et al. Organochlorine pesticides and polychlorinated biphenyl residues in foodstuffs and human tissues from china: status of contamination, historical trend, and human dietary exposure. *Arch Environ Contam Toxicol* 2002;43:473-480.

(38) Peng J, Peng L, Stevenson FF, Doctrow SR, Andersen JK. Iron and paraquat as synergistic environmental risk factors in sporadic Parkinson's disease accelerate age-related neurodegeneration. *J Neurosci* 2007;27:6914-6922.

(39) Reed L, Buchner V, Tchounwou PB. Environmental toxicology and health effects associated with hexachlorobenzene exposure. *Rev Environ Health* 2007;22:213-243.

(40) Rivas A, Cerrillo I, Granada A, Mariscal-Arcas M, Olea-Serrano F. Pesticide exposure of two age groups of women and its relationship with their diet. *Sci Total Environ* 2007;382:14-21.

(41) Tryphonas H. The impact of PCBs and dioxins on children's health: immunological considerations. *Can J Public Health* 1998;89 Suppl 1:S49-7.

(42) Tsydenova OV, Sudaryanto A, Kajiwara N, Kunisue T, Batoev VB, Tanabe S. Organohalogen compounds in human breast milk from Republic of Buryatia, Russia. *Environ Pollut* 2007;146:225-232.

(43) Viquez OM, Valentine HL, Friedman DB, Olson SJ, Valentine WM. Peripheral nerve protein expression and carbonyl content in N,N-diethlydithiocarbamate myelinopathy. *Chem Res Toxicol* 2007;20:370-379.

(44) Wade MG, Parent S, Finnson KW et al. Thyroid toxicity due to subchronic exposure to a complex mixture of 16 organochlorines, lead, and cadmium. *Toxicol Sci* 2002;67:207-218.

(45) Waliszewski SM, Pardio VT, Waliszewski KN et al. Organochlorine pesticide residues in cow's milk and butter in Mexico. *Sci Total Environ* 1997;208:127-132.

(46) Weiss J, Papke O, Bergman A. A worldwide survey of polychlorinated dibenzo-p-dioxins, dibenzofurans, and related contaminants in butter. *Ambio* 2005;34:589-597.

(47) Bloom MS, Vena JE, Swanson MK, Moysich KB, Olson JR. Profiles of ortho-polychlorinated biphenyl congeners, dichlorodiphenyldichloroethylene, hexachlorobenzene, and Mirex among male Lake Ontario sportfish consumers: the New York State Angler cohort study. *Environ Res* 2005;97:178-194.

(48) Carpy SA, Kobel W, Doe J. Health risk of low-dose pesticides mixtures: a review of the 1985-1998 literature on combination toxicology and health risk assessment. *J Toxicol Environ Health B Crit Rev* 2000;3:1-25.

(49) Swirsky GL, Stern BR, Slone TH, Brown JP, Manley NB, Ames BN. Pesticide residues in food: investigation of disparities in cancer risk estimates. *Cancer Lett* 1997;117:195-207.

(50) Gammon DW, Aldous CN, Carr WC, Jr., Sanborn JR, Pfeifer KF. A risk assessment of atrazine use in California: human health and ecological aspects. *Pest Manag Sci* 2005;61:331-355.

(51) Mao H, Fang X, Floyd KM, Polcz JE, Zhang P, Liu B. Induction of microglial reactive oxygen species production by the organochlorinated pesticide dieldrin. *Brain Res* 2007;1186:267-274.

(52) Abhilash PC, Singh N. Pesticide use and application: an Indian scenario. *J Hazard Mater* 2009;165:1-12.

(53) Gupta PK. Pesticide exposure--Indian scene. *Toxicology* 2004;198:83-90.

(54) Moser VC, Simmons JE, Gennings C. Neurotoxicological interactions of a five-pesticide mixture in preweanling rats. *Toxicol Sci* 2006;92:235-245.

(55) Boyd CA, Weiler MH, Porter WP. Behavioral and neurochemical changes associated with chronic exposure to low-level concentration of pesticide mixtures. *J Toxicol Environ Health* 1990;30:209-221.

(56) Porter WP, Green SM, Debbink NL, Carlson I. Groundwater pesticides: interactive effects of low concentrations of carbamates aldicarb and methomyl and the triazine metribuzin on thyroxine and somatotropin levels in white rats. *J Toxicol Environ Health* 1993;40:15-34.

(57) Porter WP, Jaeger JW, Carlson IH. Endocrine, immune, and behavioral effects of aldicarb (carbamate), atrazine (triazine) and nitrate (fertilizer) mixtures at groundwater concentrations. *Toxicol Ind Health* 1999;15:133-150.

(58) Thiruchelvam M, Richfield EK, Baggs RB, Tank AW, Cory-Slechta DA. The nigrostriatal dopaminergic system as a preferential target of repeated exposures to combined paraquat and maneb: implications for Parkinson's disease. *J Neurosci* 2000;20:9207-9214.

(59) Charlier C, Albert A, Herman P et al. Breast cancer and serum organochlorine residues. *Occup Environ Med* 2003;60:348-351.

(60) Brucker-Davis F, Wagner-Mahler K, Delattre I et al. Cryptorchidism at birth in Nice area (France) is associated with higher prenatal exposure to PCBs and DDE, as assessed by colostrum concentrations. *Hum Reprod* 2008;23:1708-1718.

(61) Noren K, Meironyte D. Certain organochlorine and organobromine contaminants in Swedish human milk in perspective of past 20-30 years. *Chemosphere* 2000;40:1111-1123.

(62) Wigle DT, Arbuckle TE, Walker M, Wade MG, Liu S, Krewski D. Environmental hazards: evidence for effects on child health. *J Toxicol Environ Health B Crit Rev* 2007;10:3-39.

(63) Stefanidou M, Maravelias C, Spiliopoulou C. Human exposure to endocrine disruptors and breast milk. *Endocr Metab Immune Disord Drug Targets* 2009;9:269-276.

(64) Magana-Gomez JA, de la Barca AM. Risk assessment of genetically modified crops for nutrition and health. *Nutr Rev* 2009;67:1-16.

(65) Pryme IF, Lembcke R. In vivo studies on possible health consequences of genetically modified food and feed--with particular regard to ingredients consisting of genetically modified plant materials. *Nutr Health* 2003;17:1-8.

(66) Dona A, Arvanitoyannis IS. Health risks of genetically modified foods. *Crit Rev Food Sci Nutr* 2009;49:164-175.

(67) Cantani A. Benefits and concerns associated with biotechnology-derived foods: can additional research reduce children health risks? *Eur Rev Med Pharmacol Sci* 2009;13:41-50.

(68) Key S, Ma JK, Drake PM. Genetically modified plants and human health. *J R Soc Med* 2008;101:290-298.

(69) Moneret-Vautrin DA. [Allergic risk and role of the Allergy Vigilance Network]. *Bull Acad Natl Med* 2007;191:807-814.

(70) Hanssen M, Marsden J. *E for Additives.* 2nd ed. London: Harper Collins, 1987.

(71) Ward NI, Soulsbury KA, Zettel VH, Colquhoun ID, Bunday S, Barnes B. The Influence of the Chemical Additive Tartrazine on the Zinc Status of Hyperactive Children: A Double-blind Placebo-controlled Study. *Journal of Nutritional & Environmental Medicine* 1990;1:51-57.

(72) Curl CL, Fenske RA, Elgethun K. Organophosphorus pesticide exposure of urban and suburban preschool children with organic and conventional diets. *Environ Health Perspect* 2003;111:377-382.

(73) Lester GE, Manthey JA, Buslig BS. Organic vs conventionally grown Rio Red whole grapefruit and juice: comparison of production inputs, market quality, consumer acceptance, and human health-bioactive compounds. *J Agric Food Chem* 2007;55:4474-4480.

(74) Worthington V. Nutritional quality of organic versus conventional fruits, vegetables, and grains. *J Altern Complement Med* 2001;7:161-173.

(75) Mitchell A. A two-year comparison of several quality and nutritional characteristics in tomatoes and peppers. *University of California (Davis Campus) website* [serial online] 2009; Accessed June 11, 2009.

(76) Carbonaro M, Mattera M, Nicoli S, Bergamo P, Cappelloni M. Modulation of antioxidant compounds in organic vs conventional fruit (peach, Prunus persica L., and pear, Pyrus communis L.). *J Agric Food Chem* 2002;50:5458-5462.

(77) Asami DK, Hong YJ, Barrett DM, Mitchell AE. Comparison of the total phenolic and ascorbic acid content of freeze-dried and air-dried marionberry, strawberry, and corn grown using conventional, organic, and sustainable agricultural practices. *J Agric Food Chem* 2003;51:1237-1241.

(78) Brandt K, Molgaard JP. Organic agriculture: does it enhance or reduce the nutritional value of plants foods? *Journal of Science and Food Agriculture* 2001;81:924-931.

Chapter Four References

(1) Fairfield KM, Fletcher RH. Vitamins for chronic disease prevention in adults: scientific review. *JAMA* 2002;287:3116-3126.

(2) Fletcher RH, Fairfield KM. Vitamins for chronic disease prevention in adults: clinical applications. *JAMA* 2002;287:3127-3129.

(3) Faloon W. Vindication for Linus Pauling. Life Extension [June]. 2011. Hollywood, FL, Life Extension Foundation.
Ref Type: Magazine Article

(4) Enstrom JE, Kanim LE, Klein MA. Vitamin C intake and mortality among a sample of the United States population. *Epidemiology* 1992;3:194-202.

(5) Losonczy KG, Harris TB, Havlik RJ. Vitamin E and vitamin C supplement use and risk of all-cause and coronary heart disease mortality in older persons: the Established Populations for Epidemiologic Studies of the Elderly. *Am J Clin Nutr* 1996;64:190-196.

(6) Nyyssonen K, Parviainen MT, Salonen R, Tuomilehto J, Salonen JT. Vitamin C deficiency and risk of myocardial infarction: prospective population study of men from eastern Finland. *BMJ* 1997;314:634-638.

(7) Giovannucci E, Stampfer MJ, Colditz GA et al. Multivitamin use, folate, and colon cancer in women in the Nurses' Health Study. *Ann Intern Med* 1998;129:517-524.

(8) Mansoor MA, Kristensen O, Hervig T et al. Plasma total homocysteine response to oral doses of folic acid and pyridoxine hydrochloride (vitamin B6) in healthy individuals. Oral doses of vitamin B6 reduce concentrations of serum folate. *Scand J Clin Lab Invest* 1999;59:139-146.

(9) Aksenov V, Long J, Lokuge S, Foster JA, Liu J, Rollo CD. Dietary amelioration of locomotor, neurotransmitter and mitochondrial aging. *Exp Biol Med (Maywood)* 2010;235:66-76.

(10) Lemon JA, Boreham DR, Rollo CD. A complex dietary supplement extends longevity of mice. *J Gerontol A Biol Sci Med Sci* 2005;60:275-279.

(11) Macchia A, Monte S, Pellegrini F et al. Omega-3 fatty acid supplementation reduces one-year risk of atrial fibrillation in patients hospitalized with myocardial infarction. *Eur J Clin Pharmacol* 2008;64:627-634.

(12) Gopinath B, Buyken AE, Flood VM, Empson M, Rochtchina E, Mitchell P. Consumption of polyunsaturated fatty acids, fish, and nuts and risk of inflammatory disease mortality. *Am J Clin Nutr* 2011;93:1073-1079.

(13) Leon H, Shibata MC, Sivakumaran S, Dorgan M, Chatterley T, Tsuyuki RT. Effect of fish oil on arrhythmias and mortality: systematic review. *BMJ* 2008;337:a2931.

(14) Marik PE, Varon J. Omega-3 dietary supplements and the risk of cardiovascular events: a systematic review. *Clin Cardiol* 2009;32:365-372.

(15) Zhao YT, Chen Q, Sun YX et al. Prevention of sudden cardiac death with omega-3 fatty acids in patients with coronary heart disease: a meta-analysis of randomized controlled trials. *Ann Med* 2009;41:301-310.

(16) Einvik G, Klemsdal TO, Sandvik L, Hjerkinn EM. A randomized clinical trial on n-3 polyunsaturated fatty acids supplementation and all-cause mortality in elderly men at high cardiovascular risk. *Eur J Cardiovasc Prev Rehabil* 2010;17:588-592.

(17) Jensen SS, Madsen MW, Lukas J, Binderup L, Bartek J. Inhibitory effects of 1alpha,25-dihydroxyvitamin D(3) on the G(1)-S phase-controlling machinery. *Mol Endocrinol* 2001;15:1370-1380.

(18) Lowe L, Hansen CM, Senaratne S, Colston KW. Mechanisms implicated in the growth regulatory effects of vitamin D compounds in breast cancer cells. *Recent Results Cancer Res* 2003;164:99-110.

(19) Swami S, Raghavachari N, Muller UR, Bao YP, Feldman D. Vitamin D growth inhibition of breast cancer cells: gene expression patterns assessed by cDNA microarray. *Breast Cancer Res Treat* 2003;80:49-62.

(20) Colston KW, Hansen CM. Mechanisms implicated in the growth regulatory effects of vitamin D in breast cancer. *Endocr Relat Cancer* 2002;9:45-59.

(21) Weitsman GE, Koren R, Zuck E, Rotem C, Liberman UA, Ravid A. Vitamin D sensitizes breast cancer cells to the action of H2O2: mitochondria as a convergence point in the death pathway. *Free Radic Biol Med* 2005;39:266-278.

(22) Welsh J. Vitamin D and breast cancer: insights from animal models. *Am J Clin Nutr* 2004;80:1721S-1724S.

(23) Grant WB. Epidemiology of disease risks in relation to vitamin D insufficiency. *Prog Biophys Mol Biol* 2006;92:65-79.

(24) Grant WB. A multicountry ecologic study of risk and risk reduction factors for prostate cancer mortality. *Eur Urol* 2004;45:271-279.

(25) Grant WB. An estimate of premature cancer mortality in the U.S. due to inadequate doses of solar ultraviolet-B radiation. *Cancer* 2002;94:1867-1875.

(26) Johnson TD. Guarding Against the Dangers of Vitamin D Deficiency. Life Extension Magazine [May]. 2007.
Ref Type: Magazine Article

(27) Holick M. Adventures in Globe-trotting. *The Vitamin D Solution*. New York: Hudson Street Press; 2010;74-98.

(28) Eichler I, Winkler R. [Effect and effectiveness of iodine brine baths in a spa]. *Wien Klin Wochenschr* 1994;106:265-271.

(29) HITZENBERGER G. [Comparative studies on the effects of the Bad Hall iodine cure in hypertensives]. *Arch Phys Ther (Leipz)* 1961;13:91-94.

(30) Klieber M, Czerwenka-Howorka K, Homan R, Pirker R. [Ergospirometric studies of circulation in healthy humans. Effect of iodine brine baths on work-induced changes in blood pressure, respiratory gas exchange and metabolic parameters]. *Med Welt* 1982;33:1123-1126.

(31) Lu HC. *Chinese Foods for Longevity.* New York: Sterling, 1990.

(32) Mikhno LE, Novikov SA. [The use of local iodobromine baths in the early sanatorium rehabilitation of myocardial infarct patients with arterial hypertension]. *Lik Sprava* 1992;89-91.

(33) Pitchford P. *Healing with Whole Foods: Oriental Traditions and Modern Nutrition.* Berkeley, CA: North Atlantic Books, 1993.

(34) Vinogradova MN, Mandrykina TA, Lavrov GK, Shchegoleva EA. [The effect of molecular-iodine baths on the central hemodynamics of patients with hypertension and ischemic heart disease]. *Vopr Kurortol Fizioter Lech Fiz Kult* 1990;15-18.

(35) Bastido WA. *Pharmacology, Therapeutics and Prescription Writing for Students and Practitioners.* 5th ed. Philadelphia: WB Saunders, 1947.

(36) McGuigan HA. *Applied Pharmacology.* St Louis, CV Mosby, 1940.

(37) Sollmann TH. *A Manual of Pharmacology and Its Applications to Therapeutics and Toxicology.* 7th ed. Philadelphia: 1948.

(38) Fazio S, Palmieri EA, Lombardi G, Biondi B. Effects of thyroid hormone on the cardiovascular system. *Recent Prog Horm Res* 2004;59:31-50.

(39) Cacace MG, Landau EM, Ramsden JJ. The Hofmeister series: salt and solvent effects on interfacial phenomena. *Q Rev Biophys* 1997;30:241-277.

(40) Hatefi Y, Hanstein WG. Solubilization of particulate proteins and nonelectrolytes by chaotropic agents. *Proc Natl Acad Sci U S A* 1969;62:1129-1136.

(41) Hoption Cann SA, van Netten JP, van NC. Iodized salt and hypertension. *Arch Intern Med* 2002;162:104-105.

(42) Hoption Cann SA. Hypothesis: dietary iodine intake in the etiology of cardiovascular disease. *J Am Coll Nutr* 2006;25:1-11.

(43) Miller ER, III, Pastor-Barriuso R, Dalal D, Riemersma RA, Appel LJ, Guallar E. Meta-analysis: high-dosage vitamin E supplementation may increase all-cause mortality. *Ann Intern Med* 2005;142:37-46.

(44) Wood T. The Case for Nutritional Supplements. *article submitted for publication* 2006.

Chapter Five References

(1) Vitamin D. *Wikipedia* [serial online] 2011; Accessed June 14, 2011.

(2) Davis W. VIamin D's Crucial Role in Cardiovascular Disease. Life Extension Magazine . 2007. Hollywood, FL, Life Extension Media.
Ref Type: Magazine Article

(3) Holick M. *The Vitamin D Solution.* New York: Hudson Street Press, 2010.

(4) Holick M. Dethroning the Cover-Up. *The Vitamin D Solution.* New York: Hudson Street Press; 2010;242-248.

(5) Jensen SS, Madsen MW, Lukas J, Binderup L, Bartek J. Inhibitory effects of 1alpha,25-dihydroxyvitamin D(3) on the G(1)-S phase-controlling machinery. *Mol Endocrinol* 2001;15:1370-1380.

(6) Lowe L, Hansen CM, Senaratne S, Colston KW. Mechanisms implicated in the growth regulatory effects of vitamin D compounds in breast cancer cells. *Recent Results Cancer Res* 2003;164:99-110.

(7) Swami S, Raghavachari N, Muller UR, Bao YP, Feldman D. Vitamin D growth inhibition of breast cancer cells: gene expression patterns assessed by cDNA microarray. *Breast Cancer Res Treat* 2003;80:49-62.

(8) Colston KW, Hansen CM. Mechanisms implicated in the growth regulatory effects of vitamin D in breast cancer. *Endocr Relat Cancer* 2002;9:45-59.

(9) Weitsman GE, Koren R, Zuck E, Rotem C, Liberman UA, Ravid A. Vitamin D sensitizes breast cancer cells to the action of H2O2: mitochondria as a convergence point in the death pathway. *Free Radic Biol Med* 2005;39:266-278.

(10) Welsh J. Vitamin D and breast cancer: insights from animal models. *Am J Clin Nutr* 2004;80:1721S-1724S.

(11) Grant WB. Epidemiology of disease risks in relation to vitamin D insufficiency. *Prog Biophys Mol Biol* 2006;92:65-79.

(12) Grant WB. A multicountry ecologic study of risk and risk reduction factors for prostate cancer mortality. *Eur Urol* 2004;45:271-279.

(13) Grant WB. An estimate of premature cancer mortality in the U.S. due to inadequate doses of solar ultraviolet-B radiation. *Cancer* 2002;94:1867-1875.

(14) Johnson TD. Guarding Against the Dangers of Vitamin D Deficiency. Life Extension Magazine [May]. 2007.
Ref Type: Magazine Article

(15) Holick M. Adventures in Globe-trotting. *The Vitamin D Solution.* New York: Hudson Street Press; 2010;74-98.

(16) Garland C, Shekelle RB, Barrett-Connor E, Criqui MH, Rossof AH, Paul O. Dietary vitamin D and calcium and risk of colorectal cancer: a 19-year prospective study in men. *Lancet* 1985;1:307-309.

(17) Gorham ED, Garland CF, Garland FC et al. Vitamin D and prevention of colorectal cancer. *J Steroid Biochem Mol Biol* 2005;97:179-194.

(18) Bakhru A, Mallinger JB, Buckanovich RJ, Griggs JJ. Casting light on 25-hydroxyvitamin D deficiency in ovarian cancer: a study from the NHANES. *Gynecol Oncol* 2010;119:314-318.

(19) Garland CF, Garland FC, Gorham ED et al. The role of vitamin D in cancer prevention. *Am J Public Health* 2006;96:252-261.

(20) Grant WB, Mohr SB. Ecological studies of ultraviolet B, vitamin D and cancer since 2000. *Ann Epidemiol* 2009;19:446-454.

(21) Grant WB. An ecological study of cancer incidence and mortality rates in France with respect to latitude, an index for vitamin D production. *Dermatoendocrinol* 2010;2:62-67.

(22) Karami S, Boffetta P, Stewart P et al. Occupational sunlight exposure and risk of renal cell carcinoma. *Cancer* 2010;116:2001-2010.

(23) Mohr SB, Garland CF, Gorham ED, Grant WB, Garland FC. Could ultraviolet B irradiance and vitamin D be associated with lower incidence rates of lung cancer? *J Epidemiol Community Health* 2008;62:69-74.

(24) Mohr SB, Garland CF, Gorham ED, Grant WB, Garland FC. Ultraviolet B irradiance and vitamin D status are inversely associated with incidence rates of pancreatic cancer worldwide. *Pancreas* 2010;39:669-674.

(25) Mohr SB, Gorham ED, Garland CF, Grant WB, Garland FC. Low ultraviolet B and increased risk of brain cancer: an ecological study of 175 countries. *Neuroepidemiology* 2010;35:281-290.

(26) Mohr SB, Garland CF, Gorham ED, Grant WB, Garland FC. Ultraviolet B and incidence rates of leukemia worldwide. *Am J Prev Med* 2011;41:68-74.

(27) Musselman JR, Spector LG. Childhood cancer incidence in relation to sunlight exposure. *Br J Cancer* 2011;104:214-220.

(28) Neale RE, Youlden DR, Krnjacki L, Kimlin MG, van der Pols JC. Latitude variation in pancreatic cancer mortality in Australia. *Pancreas* 2009;38:387-390.

(29) Oh EY, Ansell C, Nawaz H, Yang CH, Wood PA, Hrushesky WJ. Global breast cancer seasonality. *Breast Cancer Res Treat* 2010;123:233-243.

(30) Pierrot-Deseilligny C, Souberbielle JC. Widespread vitamin D insufficiency: A new challenge for primary prevention, with particular reference to multiple sclerosis. *Presse Med* 2011;40:349-356.

(31) Lappe JM, Travers-Gustafson D, Davies KM, Recker RR, Heaney RP. Vitamin D and calcium supplementation reduces cancer risk: results of a randomized trial. *Am J Clin Nutr* 2007;85:1586-1591.

(32) Scragg R, Jackson R, Holdaway IM, Lim T, Beaglehole R. Myocardial infarction is inversely associated with plasma 25-hydroxyvitamin D3 levels: a community-based study. *Int J Epidemiol* 1990;19:559-563.

(33) Spencer FA, Goldberg RJ, Becker RC, Gore JM. Seasonal distribution of acute myocardial infarction in the second National Registry of Myocardial Infarction. *J Am Coll Cardiol* 1998;31:1226-1233.

(34) Ku CS, Yang CY, Lee WJ, Chiang HT, Liu CP, Lin SL. Absence of a seasonal variation in myocardial infarction onset in a region without temperature extremes. *Cardiology* 1998;89:277-282.

(35) Grimes DS, Hindle E, Dyer T. Sunlight, cholesterol and coronary heart disease. *QJM* 1996;89:579-589.

(36) Giovannucci E, Liu Y, Hollis BW, Rimm EB. 25-hydroxyvitamin D and risk of myocardial infarction in men: a prospective study. *Arch Intern Med* 2008;168:1174-1180.

(37) Lind L, Hanni A, Lithell H, Hvarfner A, Sorensen OH, Ljunghall S. Vitamin D is related to blood pressure and other cardiovascular risk factors in middle-aged men. *Am J Hypertens* 1995;8:894-901.

(38) Martins D, Wolf M, Pan D et al. Prevalence of cardiovascular risk factors and the serum levels of 25-hydroxyvitamin D in the United States: data from the Third National Health and Nutrition Examination Survey. *Arch Intern Med* 2007;167:1159-1165.

(39) Pfeifer M, Begerow B, Minne HW, Nachtigall D, Hansen C. Effects of a short-term vitamin D(3) and calcium supplementation on blood pressure and parathyroid hormone levels in elderly women. *J Clin Endocrinol Metab* 2001;86:1633-1637.

(40) Timms PM, Mannan N, Hitman GA et al. Circulating MMP9, vitamin D and variation in the TIMP-1 response with VDR genotype: mechanisms for inflammatory damage in chronic disorders? *QJM* 2002;95:787-796.

(41) Davis W. Vitamin D's Crucial Role in Cardiovascular Protection. Life Extension Magazine [September]. 2007. Ref Type: Magazine Article

(42) Achinger SG, Ayus JC. The role of vitamin D in left ventricular hypertrophy and cardiac function. *Kidney Int Suppl* 2005;S37-S42.

(43) London GM, Guerin AP, Verbeke FH et al. Mineral metabolism and arterial functions in end-stage renal disease: potential role of 25-hydroxyvitamin D deficiency. *J Am Soc Nephrol* 2007;18:613-620.

(44) Zittermann A, Schleithoff SS, Tenderich G, Berthold HK, Korfer R, Stehle P. Low vitamin D status: a contributing factor in the pathogenesis of congestive heart failure? *J Am Coll Cardiol* 2003;41:105-112.

(45) Lindqvist PG, Epstein E, Olsson H. Does an active sun exposure habit lower the risk of venous thrombotic events? A D-lightful hypothesis. *J Thromb Haemost* 2009;7:605-610.

(46) Schleithoff SS, Zittermann A, Tenderich G, Berthold HK, Stehle P, Koerfer R. Vitamin D supplementation improves cytokine profiles in patients with congestive heart failure: a double-blind, randomized, placebo-controlled trial. *Am J Clin Nutr* 2006;83:754-759.

(47) Kiefer D. Why is flu risk so much higher in the winter? Life Extension Magazine [February], 22-28. 2007. Life Extension Media.
Ref Type: Magazine Article

(48) Lochner JD, Schneider DJ. [The relationship between tuberculosis, vitamin D, potassium and AIDS. A message for South Africa?]. *S Afr Med J* 1994;84:79-82.

(49) Bellamy R, Ruwende C, Corrah T et al. Tuberculosis and chronic hepatitis B virus infection in Africans and variation in the vitamin D receptor gene. *J Infect Dis* 1999;179:721-724.

(50) Schauber J, Dorschner RA, Coda AB et al. Injury enhances TLR2 function and antimicrobial peptide expression through a vitamin D-dependent mechanism. *J Clin Invest* 2007;117:803-811.

(51) Strohle A, Wolters M, Hahn A. Micronutrients at the interface between inflammation and infection--ascorbic acid and calciferol. Part 2: calciferol and the significance of nutrient supplements. *Inflamm Allergy Drug Targets* 2011;10:64-74.

(52) Hoeck AD, Pall ML. Will vitamin D supplementation ameliorate diseases characterized by chronic inflammation and fatigue? *Med Hypotheses* 2011;76:208-213.

(53) Sundar IK, Hwang JW, Wu S, Sun J, Rahman I. Deletion of vitamin D receptor leads to premature emphysema/COPD by increased matrix metalloproteinases and lymphoid aggregates formation. *Biochem Biophys Res Commun* 2011;406:127-133.

(54) Bahar-Shany K, Ravid A, Koren R. Upregulation of MMP-9 production by TNFalpha in keratinocytes and its attenuation by vitamin D. *J Cell Physiol* 2010;222:729-737.

(55) Holick M. Supplement Safely. *The Vitamin D Solution*. New York: Hudson Street Press; 2010;212-228.

(56) Miller DW. Iodine For Health. *www lewrockwell com* [serial online] 2006; Accessed June 26, 2012.

(57) Crockford SJ. Evolutionary roots of iodine and thyroid hormones in cell-cell signaling. *Integr Comp Biol* 2009;49:155-166.

(58) Hunt S. Halogenated tyrosine derivatives in invertebrate scleroproteins: isolation and identification. In: Wold F, Moldave K, eds. *Methods in Enzymology*. Volume 107 Postrsanslational Modifications Part B ed. New York: Academic Press; 1984;413-438.

(59) Poncin S, Gerard AC, Boucquey M et al. Oxidative stress in the thyroid gland: from harmlessness to hazard depending on the iodine content. *Endocrinology* 2008;149:424-433.

(60) Pizzorno L. Iodine: The Next Vitamin D? Part II. *Logevity Medicine Review* [serial online] 2012.

(61) Venturi S. Is there a role for iodine in breast diseases? *Breast* 2001;10:379-382.

(62) Patrick L. Iodine: deficiency and therapeutic considerations. *Altern Med Rev* 2008;13:116-127.

(63) Higdon J. Iodine. Linus Pauling Institute . 2010. 4-6-2012.
Ref Type: Video Recording

(64) DeLong GR, Leslie PW, Wang SH et al. Effect on infant mortality of iodination of irrigation water in a severely iodine-deficient area of China. *Lancet* 1997;350:771-773.

(65) Haddow JE, Palomaki GE, Allan WC et al. Maternal thyroid deficiency during pregnancy and subsequent neuropsychological development of the child. *N Engl J Med* 1999;341:549-555.

(66) Klein RZ, Sargent JD, Larsen PR, Waisbren SE, Haddow JE, Mitchell ML. Relation of severity of maternal hypothyroidism to cognitive development of offspring. *J Med Screen* 2001;8:18-20.

(67) Vermiglio F, Lo P, V, Moleti M et al. Attention deficit and hyperactivity disorders in the offspring of mothers exposed to mild-moderate iodine deficiency: a possible novel iodine deficiency disorder in developed countries. *J Clin Endocrinol Metab* 2004;89:6054-6060.

(68) Hoption Cann SA. Hypothesis: dietary iodine intake in the etiology of cardiovascular disease. *J Am Coll Nutr* 2006;25:1-11.

(69) Biondi B, Klein I. Hypothyroidism as a risk factor for cardiovascular disease. *Endocrine* 2004;24:1-13.

(70) Dillmann WH. Cellular action of thyroid hormone on the heart. *Thyroid* 2002;12:447-452.

(71) Flechas JD. Orthoiodosupplementation in a Prmary Care Practice. *The Orginal Internist* 2005;89-96.

(72) Wiseman RA. Breast cancer hypothesis: a single cause for the majority of cases. *J Epidemiol Community Health* 2000;54:851-858.

(73) Abraham GE. The safe and effective implementation of orthoiodosupplemenation in medical practice. *The Original Internist* 2005;112-118.

(74) Derry D. *Breast Cancer and Iodine*. Victoria, BC: Trafford Publishing, 2001.

(75) Eskin BA. Iodine and mammary cancer. *Adv Exp Med Biol* 1977;91:293-304.

(76) Ghent WR, Eskin BA, Low DA, Hill LP. Iodine replacement in fibrocystic disease of the breast. *Can J Surg* 1993;36:453-460.

(77) Stadel BV. Dietary iodine and risk of breast, endometrial, and ovarian cancer. *Lancet* 1976;1:890-891.

(78) Eskin BA, Bartuska DG, Dunn MR, Jacob G, Dratman MB. Mammary gland dysplasia in iodine deficiency. Studies in rats. *JAMA* 1967;200:691-695.

(79) Smyth PP. Thyroid disease and breast cancer. *J Endocrinol Invest* 1993;16:396-401.

(80) Miller DW. Extrathyroidal Benefits of Iodine. *J Am Phys Surg* 2006;11:106-110.

(81) Zhang L, Sharma S, Zhu LX et al. Nonradioactive iodide effectively induces apoptosis in genetically modified lung cancer cells. *Cancer Res* 2003;63:5065-5072.

(82) Sekiya M, Funahashi H, Tsukamura K et al. Intracellular signaling in the induction of apoptosis in a human breast cancer cell line by water extract of Mekabu. *Int J Clin Oncol* 2005;10:122-126.

(83) Shrivastava A, Tiwari M, Sinha RA et al. Molecular iodine induces caspase-independent apoptosis in human breast carcinoma cells involving the mitochondria-mediated pathway. *J Biol Chem* 2006;281:19762-19771.

(84) Golkowski F, Szybinski Z, Rachtan J et al. Iodine prophylaxis--the protective factor against stomach cancer in iodine deficient areas. *Eur J Nutr* 2007;46:251-256.

(85) Abnet CC, Fan JH, Kamangar F et al. Self-reported goiter is associated with a significantly increased risk of gastric noncardia adenocarcinoma in a large population-based Chinese cohort. *Int J Cancer* 2006;119:1508-1510.

(86) Burgess JR, Dwyer T, McArdle K, Tucker P, Shugg D. The changing incidence and spectrum of thyroid carcinoma in Tasmania (1978-1998) during a transition from iodine sufficiency to iodine deficiency. *J Clin Endocrinol Metab* 2000;85:1513-1517.

(87) Franceschi S, Preston-Martin S, Dal ML et al. A pooled analysis of case-control studies of thyroid cancer. IV. Benign thyroid diseases. *Cancer Causes Control* 1999;10:583-595.

(88) Mellemgaard A, From G, Jorgensen T, Johansen C, Olsen JH, Perrild H. Cancer risk in individuals with benign thyroid disorders. *Thyroid* 1998;8:751-754.

(89) Schaller RT, Jr., Stevenson JK. Development of carcinoma of the thyroid in iodine-deficient mice. *Cancer* 1966;19:1063-1080.

(90) Shakhtarin VV, Tsyb AF, Stepanenko VF, Orlov MY, Kopecky KJ, Davis S. Iodine deficiency, radiation dose, and the risk of thyroid cancer among children and adolescents in the Bryansk region of Russia following the Chernobyl power station accident. *Int J Epidemiol* 2003;32:584-591.

(91) Eichler I, Winkler R. [Effect and effectiveness of iodine brine baths in a spa]. *Wien Klin Wochenschr* 1994;106:265-271.

(92) HITZENBERGER G. [Comparative studies on the effects of the Bad Hall iodine cure in hypertensives]. *Arch Phys Ther (Leipz)* 1961;13:91-94.

(93) Klieber M, Czerwenka-Howorka K, Homan R, Pirker R. [Ergospirometric studies of circulation in healthy humans. Effect of iodine brine baths on work-induced changes in blood pressure, respiratory gas exchange and metabolic parameters]. *Med Welt* 1982;33:1123-1126.

(94) Lu HC. *Chinese Foods for Longevity*. New York: Sterling, 1990.

(95) Mikhno LE, Novikov SA. [The use of local iodobromine baths in the early sanatorium rehabilitation of myocardial infarct patients with arterial hypertension]. *Lik Sprava* 1992;89-91.

(96) Pitchford P. *Healing with Whole Foods: Oriental Traditions and Modern Nutrition*. Berkeley, CA: North Atlantic Books, 1993.

(97) Vinogradova MN, Mandrykina TA, Lavrov GK, Shchegoleva EA. [The effect of molecular-iodine baths on the central hemodynamics of patients with hypertension and ischemic heart disease]. *Vopr Kurortol Fizioter Lech Fiz Kult* 1990;15-18.

(98) Bastido WA. *Pharmacology, Therapeutics and Prescription Writing for Students and Practitioners.* 5th ed. Philadelphia: WB Saunders, 1947.

(99) McGuigan HA. *Applied Pharmacology.* St Louis, CV Mosby, 1940.

(100) Sollmann TH. *A Manual of Pharmacology and Its Applications to Therapeutics and Toxicology.* 7th ed. Philadelphia: 1948.

(101) Fazio S, Palmieri EA, Lombardi G, Biondi B. Effects of thyroid hormone on the cardiovascular system. *Recent Prog Horm Res* 2004;59:31-50.

(102) Cacace MG, Landau EM, Ramsden JJ. The Hofmeister series: salt and solvent effects on interfacial phenomena. *Q Rev Biophys* 1997;30:241-277.

(103) Hatefi Y, Hanstein WG. Solubilization of particulate proteins and nonelectrolytes by chaotropic agents. *Proc Natl Acad Sci U S A* 1969;62:1129-1136.

(104) Hoption Cann SA, van Netten JP, van NC. Iodized salt and hypertension. *Arch Intern Med* 2002;162:104-105.

(105) Canturk Z, Cetinarslan B, Tarkun I, Canturk NZ, Ozden M. Lipid profile and lipoprotein (a) as a risk factor for cardiovascular disease in women with subclinical hypothyroidism. *Endocr Res* 2003;29:307-316.

(106) Kahaly GJ. Cardiovascular and atherogenic aspects of subclinical hypothyroidism. *Thyroid* 2000;10:665-679.

(107) Park YJ, Lee YJ, Choi SI, Chun EJ, Jang HC, Chang HJ. Impact of subclinical hypothyroidism on the coronary artery disease in apparently healthy subjects. *Eur J Endocrinol* 2011;165:115-121.

(108) Haentjens P, Van MA, Poppe K, Velkeniers B. Subclinical thyroid dysfunction and mortality: an estimate of relative and absolute excess all-cause mortality based on time-to-event data from cohort studies. *Eur J Endocrinol* 2008;159:329-341.

(109) Auer J, Berent R, Weber T, Lassnig E, Eber B. Thyroid function is associated with presence and severity of coronary atherosclerosis. *Clin Cardiol* 2003;26:569-573.

(110) Bruckert E, Giral P, Chadarevian R, Turpin G. Low free-thyroxine levels are a risk factor for subclinical atherosclerosis in euthyroid hyperlipidemic patients. *J Cardiovasc Risk* 1999;6:327-331.

(111) Dagre AG, Lekakis JP, Protogerou AD et al. Abnormal endothelial function in female patients with hypothyroidism and borderline thyroid function. *Int J Cardiol* 2007;114:332-338.

(112) Yun KH, Jeong MH, Oh SK et al. Relationship of thyroid stimulating hormone with coronary atherosclerosis in angina patients. *Int J Cardiol* 2007;122:56-60.

(113) Cappola AR, Ladenson PW. Hypothyroidism and atherosclerosis. *J Clin Endocrinol Metab* 2003;88:2438-2444.

(114) den Hollander JG, Wulkan RW, Mantel MJ, Berghout A. Correlation between severity of thyroid dysfunction and renal function. *Clin Endocrinol (Oxf)* 2005;62:423-427.

(115) Klein I, Danzi S. Thyroid disease and the heart. *Circulation* 2007;116:1725-1735.

(116) Muller B, Tsakiris DA, Roth CB, Guglielmetti M, Staub JJ, Marbet GA. Haemostatic profile in hypothyroidism as potential risk factor for vascular or thrombotic disease. *Eur J Clin Invest* 2001;31:131-137.

(117) Tomanek RJ, Busch TL. Coordinated capillary and myocardial growth in response to thyroxine treatment. *Anat Rec* 1998;251:44-49.

(118) Iqbal A, Jorde R, Figenschau Y. Serum lipid levels in relation to serum thyroid-stimulating hormone and the effect of thyroxine treatment on serum lipid levels in subjects with subclinical hypothyroidism: the Tromso Study. *J Intern Med* 2006;260:53-61.

(119) Rizos CV, Elisaf MS, Liberopoulos EN. Effects of thyroid dysfunction on lipid profile. *Open Cardiovasc Med J* 2011;5:76-84.

(120) American Cancer Society. Benign Breast Conditions. *cancer org* [serial online] 2001.

(121) Brownstein D. Clinical Experience with Inorganic, Non-radioactive Iodine/Iodide. *The Original Internist* 2005;105-108.

(122) Pizzorno L. Iodine: the Next Vitamin D? Part II. *Longevity Medicine Review* [serial online] 2010; Accessed November 7, 2012.

(123) Smyth PP. Role of iodine in antioxidant defence in thyroid and breast disease. *Biofactors* 2003;19:121-130.

(124) Bretthauer EW, Mullen AL, Moghissi AA. Milk transfer comparisons of different chemical forms of radioiodine. *Health Phys* 1972;22:257-260.

(125) Piccone N. The Silent Epidemic of Iodine Deficiency. Life Extension Magazine October. 2011.
Ref Type: Magazine Article

(126) Dunn JT. Seven deadly sins in confronting endemic iodine deficiency, and how to avoid them. *J Clin Endocrinol Metab* 1996;81:1332-1335.

(127) World Health Organization. Iodine Deficiency Disorders: Fact Sheet No. 121. 1996. Geneva, Switzerland, World Health Organization.
Ref Type: Pamphlet

(128) Triggiani V, Tafaro E, Giagulli VA et al. Role of iodine, selenium and other micronutrients in thyroid function and disorders. *Endocr Metab Immune Disord Drug Targets* 2009;9:277-294.

Lyle MacWilliam, MSc, FP
President, *NutriSearch* Corporation

Author, educator and biochemist, Lyle MacWilliam is president and CEO of NutriSearch Corporation, a Canadian research company serving the needs of the natural health products industry in the global marketplace.

A scientific consultant and public advocate for the supplement industry, Mr. MacWilliam's research and communication skills have been solicited by several agencies. Mr. MacWilliam served at the behest of Canada's former Minister of Health as a member of an expert advisory team charged with developing an innovative framework to ensure Canadians have access to safe, effective and high quality natural health products. He has also served as a management consultant with Health Canada, Environment Canada, Human Resources Development Canada, and the British Columbia Science Council, and he has been engaged as a scientific consultant for nutritional manufacturers in the United States, Canada and Mexico.

Mr. MacWilliam has served as a contributory writer for Life Extension Foundation, a US-based non-profit agency dedicated to the scientific exploration of optimal health and longevity. His creative works, including the popular *NutriSearch Comparative Guide to Nutritional Supplements*,™ are available in English, Spanish, French and Chinese. They are used by leading nutritional manufacturers, healthcare professionals and informed consumers alike, as reliable evidence-based tools with which to sort through the maze of nutritional supplements in the market today. Mr. MacWilliam is a member of the Society of Industry leaders, an international organization dedicated to bringing together authorities from all fields in a global network connecting industry veterans and academia professionals with institutional investors.

A former Canadian Member of Parliament and Member of the Legislative Assembly for British Columbia, Mr. MacWilliam is also an accomplished martial artist with a passionate commitment to personal fitness and health. His written works hit hard at today's lifestyle and dietary patterns and their role in the development of degenerative disease. His scientifically rigorous, no-nonsense delivery—served with a touch of humour—has earned him praise internationally as a sought-after speaker on the importance of optimal nutrition and lifestyle in preventive health.

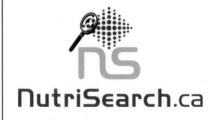